AF256304

STATUTORY VAPE

STATUTORY VAPE

*How the e-cigarette Industry Addicted a
New Generation of Youth*

JENNIFER BANMILLER AND WILSON TSAI, MD

Copyright © 2020 Wingtip Communications Inc.

All rights reserved.

No part of this book may be reproduced, or stored in a retrieval system, or transmitted in any form or by any means, electronic, mechanical, photocopying, recording, or otherwise, without express written permission of the publisher.

Published by Periscope Group, Danville, CA

www.periscopegroup.com

ISBN 978-1-7334315-2-1

First Edition

Printed in the United States of America

Table of Contents

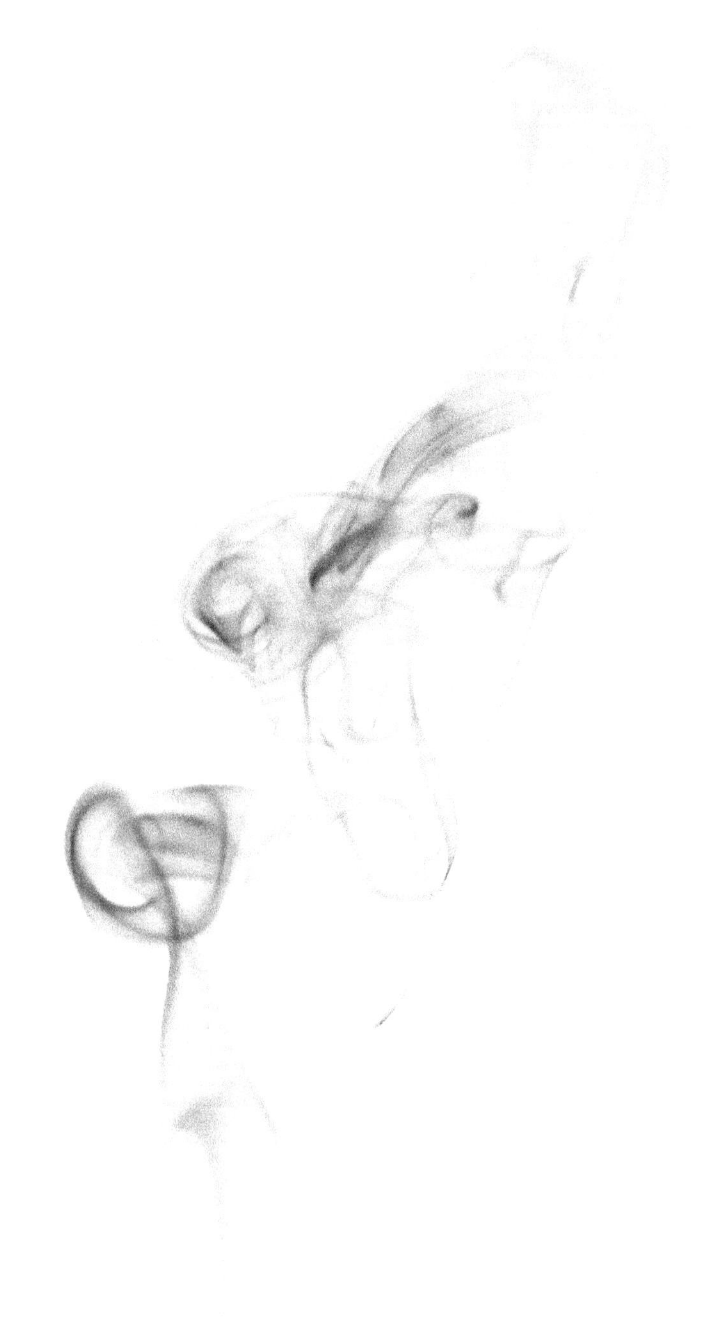

PREFACE

"Death snatches away many blooming children, the only hopes of their doting parents: how many ... have been one day in the bloom of health and hope, and the next a prey?"

—— MARY SHELLEY, *FRANKENSTEIN*

I had just finished the book *Crystal Mesh* — the unconscionable story of how women's vital health concerns were routinely traded for increased profits by some of the world's most well-known medical device makers, and woefully abetted by our broken medical regulatory review system here in the U.S. It was an exhausting project because as part of my work I had been watching up-close the physical and emotional carnage it had caused for women for eight years. Readers wrote to us and shared their profound sadness that it was all so unnecessary, that these women and their families did not need to be injured, that the system had failed them so miserably, and that it had happened in broad daylight right under all our noses, with the entire medical/technology ecosystem marching together in lock step, until finally the horror became clear to all.

And here we are again. The parallels are stunning and maddening. This time it is Big Tobacco – AGAIN – and other high-tech vaping purveyors, rather than the medical device makers at the heart of the vaginal mesh scandal. But the playbook is the same: Build seemingly attractive products which at their heart are untested and often downright dangerous, market them using huge financial resources and effective audience targeting techniques, and keep the FDA and legislators in the dark or on your side to make sure you don't have any interference as you scale your business to massive revenue opportunities. And when the whole thing blows up (and it always eventually does), never admit guilt or say you are sorry, and never pay out to the consumer early. Let them be so exhausted and in debt from medical bills that they'll take anything. The huge losers in these stories of corporate greed and malpractice are always regular people (and taxpayers) who trusted the system and believed the hype, and end up hurt – and it is so painful to realize, sometimes even dead – in the end.

Like many others, I knew that vaping was akin to smoking cigarettes without the awful tar of tobacco, but no one seemed to realize, especially the child victims and their families, that in addition to the strong addictive elements, how the chemical vapors themselves can literally light your insides on fire like a wild arsonist on the loose inside your lungs. Such critical facts were conveniently ignored in the all-out marketing blitz. These new provocative vaping products are the Jeffrey Epstein of tobacco products — they prey on the underaged and the vulnerable.

When the reports of vape victims in the thousands starting surfacing, I met with experts like Dr. Wilson Tsai who really understood the scientific issues and the great danger at play for so many millions of consumers around the world.

These companies were shamelessly funding summer camps for elementary school kids, paying community and church groups to distribute their material to their members, and targeting veterans group and other vulnerable populations. They were using their huge financial resources to build a growing market, hooking their customers for life even as they shortened the lives of those very customers, eerily reminiscent of Big Tobacco's actions with cigarettes throughout the prior decades.

It has been predatory, it was premeditated as part of a business strategy, and the greatest harm has fallen on our most vulnerable — our children. It was certainly possible to focus entirely on the over-21 adult market and still have a huge potential marketplace, but the greed impulse was just too strong (again) and the children were such a huge and impressionable audience.

And now we as a society are paying that huge price — a public health crisis bigger than any our country has faced in decades, stealing children's health and youth and leaving families in despair.

Vaping Transmitted Diseases — VTDs — are actually growing faster than STDs at an alarming rate in U.S children. But the public never really saw it coming until very recently when the many staggering stories of these vaping-related illnesses literally exploded onto the scene.

Vaping is akin to setting your internal organs on fire the minute you do it — whether that's once, twice or many times. And BOOM – life as you and your family know it can be over immediately. Immediately. No warning. Boom. Just Boom.

And that is why we are writing this book. To help bring some perspective and information to this critical, still-unfolding, and all-too-avoidable adolescent public health crisis. Vaping is smoking. Vaping is using drugs. Vaping is dangerous. Vaping could kill you.

Stop being suckers. Protect your kids. And kids, if you want to have any kind of life — glamorous, meaningful or long — this popular pastime called vaping is going to rip that dream from you.

Jennifer Banmiller
Danville, California

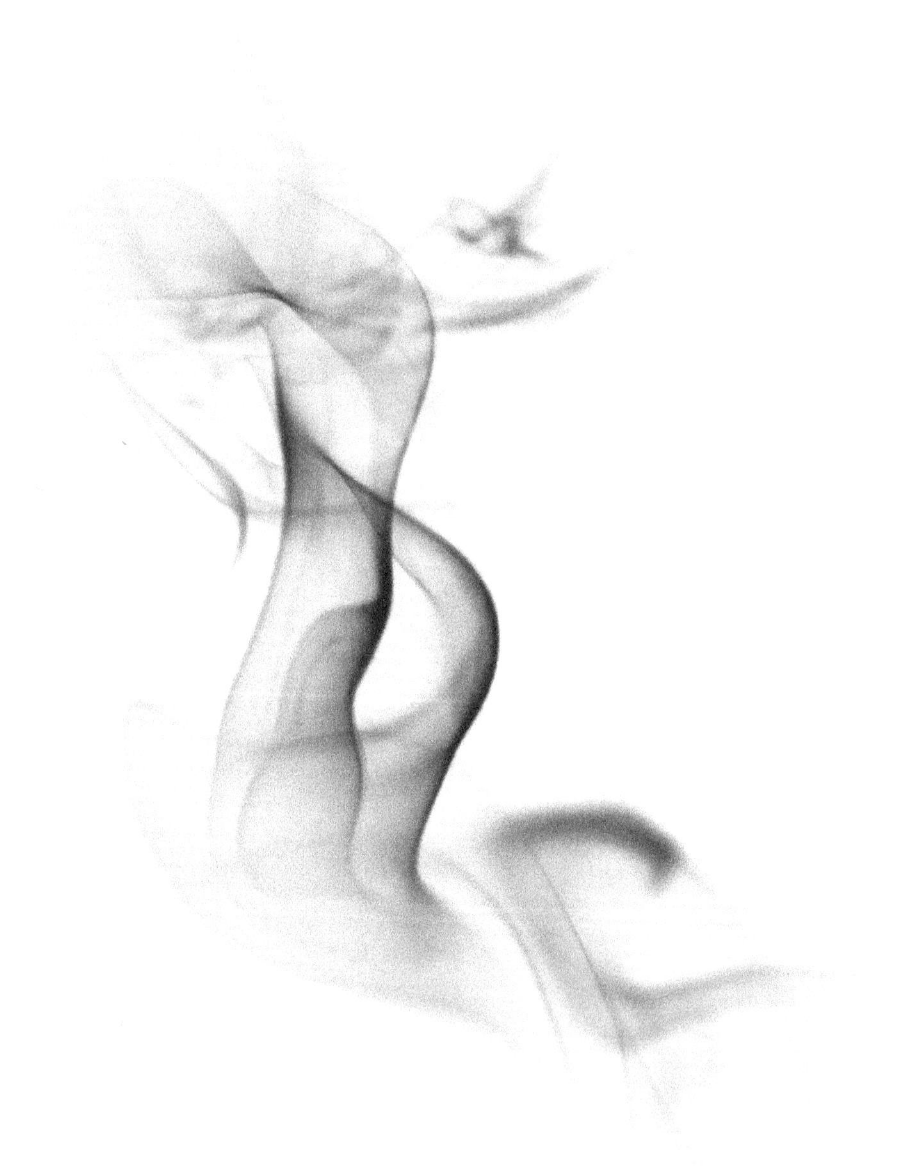

INTRODUCTION

At the time this book was published, the CDC reported that there were 64 deaths confirmed in 27 states and the District of Columbia due to vaping-related illnesses. In addition, 2,758 cases of EVALI (e-cigarette or Vaping Product Use Associated Lung Injury) hospitalization cases or deaths had been reported nationwide.

We expect this count to grow significantly as these numbers reflect only cases where vaping was the certain culprit. Many hospitalizations, catastrophic injuries and deaths have not yet been reported as tied to vaping, because at the time of admittance and diagnosis, medical doctors and health facilities were not yet aware of this direct cause. Since the CDC started defining the symptoms and reporting the numbers in September 2019, the rate of incidences has continued to climb. If you as a reader wish to be informed about the most recent data as this public health tragedy continues to unfold, please go to www.statutoryvape.com for updates.

Is anyone listening?

This photograph below is from a gas station down the street from my office. Even after the recent ban on certain cartridge flavors, when I asked the owner what flavors he had, sure enough there were still some banned flavors available because the law allows merchants to deplete their stocks. Yet he confirmed that no local parents or neighboring business owners had protested in any way or asked him to stop selling these incredibly destructive products. In order to stem the tide of this growing teen health disaster, parents, families, friends, and local businesses and authorities will all need to be involved. Vaping is an epidemic and it is killing kids in broad daylight. It will take a village to stop it.

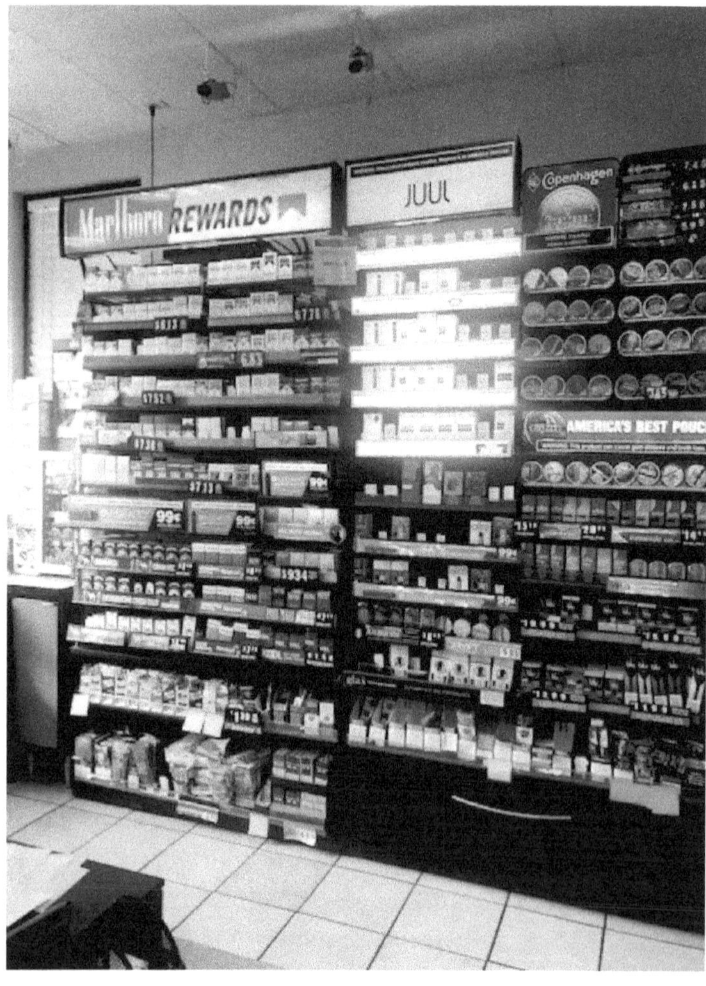

CHAPTER 1

Profiling the Vapist

When do you think the founders of Juul knew that they were systematically killing children in a no less brutal way and in vastly greater numbers than a shooter at a high school?

Was it when they...

- Secured the documents from big tobacco firms that described exactly how to create addiction?

- Discovered that it was more profitable to addict children instead of adults?

- Used that information to create a marketing strategy and action plan to addict children?

- Added the MOST addictive concentrations to the capsules to maximize and expedite addiction?

- Designed the smallest and sleekest techie product that could easily be hidden from parents?

- Flooded social media to recruit and target youth as young as 11 (middle school)?

- Circumvented scrutiny and investigation with misrepresentation and took steps to placate rather than definitively reduce harm?

- Ignored the strokes, seizures, heart attacks, overdoses, suicides and deaths?

Wolf in sheep's clothing?

In fact, the founders, makers, and investors in Juul not only ignored the risks and perils experienced by users of their products, but failed to warn the public of any potential hazards, and systematically sought to minimize and divert the scrutiny on the damages with misrepresentation, more and better legal denials and continued marketing strategies.

Why? When obvious attention to the negative effects, harm, and addiction, especially in youth was being discovered and uncovered, why would Juul continue to make and market their e-cigarettes? Only one reason: money. The product went from a rudimentary college thesis to a 38-billion-dollar company in under fifteen years. Money trumped the health of the country's youth. Money and greed are the culprits that perpetrated these vicious crimes. Here's how:

In 2004 graduate students Adam Bowen and James Monsees created a master's thesis and video that they hoped would revolutionize the smoking industry. In the video, using a combination of facts and humor, they presented their case for the creation of a non-addictive and non-combustible cigarette. The prototype for a seemingly-harmless alternative to smoking is offered to smokers looking for a safe and socially acceptable product that will reduce health risks, social shaming and isolation. It's very well received. https://www.youtube.com/watch?v=ZBDLqWCjsMM&has_verified=1

Using words like "inexpensive," "durable," and "elegant," the presenters almost breezily dismiss the "gas problems" in a typical cigarette, stating that with the liquid in their prototype "there's none of that." They go on to say that in real-life test settings it seemed like a light and healthy alternative to users. Only with a minute left in their presentation is there talk of safety, in the form of a brief mention of studies in the lab but no testing on any subjects, animal or human. There is mention of further testing they'd like to do. However, the emphasis is on design, elegance, luxury, and the "nicotine and flavor" pods are compared to Nespresso coffee pods. Can you say "marketing"? Let the packaging games begin.

Over the next few years, in various interviews with Bowen and Monsees, it becomes apparent that, contrary to their 2019 claims about their intent to deliver a less harmful cigarette, a driving goal for their e-cigarette production was to reduce more of the behavioral disadvantages of smoking, specifically "fear of being seen with a cigarette, frequent trips outside in the cold, and paranoia about smelling of smoke on a first date." *Stanford Magazine, 2012*. And, "convinced they could not only eliminate these negatives, but also build a more enjoyable experience around tobacco, the designers drew inspiration from hookahs and coffee pods. Their first prototypes were ad-hoc assemblies of bespoke components and items found on drugstore shelves. Lighters were cracked open and connected to small tobacco-filled chambers."

Vaping is smoking!

In fact, as the friends launch their company, PLOOM, and their first product, PAX, most interviews about the details of the product focused on solving the problems of taste, second-hand smoke in terms of smell, the "experience" and social acceptance. There is mention of the science behind the product, some of its components and its heating mechanism, but not safety.

"Smoking is in a different category," Monsees states, in an interview with socialunderground.com.

"It has the capability of always being luxurious, always being sort of a wonderful experience. The products that were on the market before then were sort of wooden boxes, weird stuff. That's fun in a sort of novelty way, right? That's fun from time to time. We want to build products that have kind of a magical consumer experience that you can have all the time and keep with you and it's sort of precious. A sort of obvious and intuitive consumer interface. And something that is really elegant and, contrary to concealment, you're sort of proud to be with it. That's what we were going after."

Maybe someone should have shown James Monsees the glamorous side of lung cancer and the magical consumer experience of a medically-induced coma.

https://socialunderground.com/2015/01/pax-ploom-origins-future-james-monsees/

Additionally, by studying what worked and what didn't for the big tobacco firms, the friends became educated, in a shockingly inverse way, of how best to lure, capture, and keep their victims, aka users, as hostages for years, till sickness or death do us part.

To let the gravity of this sink in, let's take a look at what was going on at the time. The big tobacco companies were involved in multiple lawsuits and the transcripts and records from the companies' archives were made surprisingly available for the first time. Documents marked "SECRET" were not only able to be perused but were even touted by Juul's founders as information that gave Juul "another leg up." Here is the actual and frightening summary of that secret memo from the same court documents available to Bowen and Monsees:

Title: Research Planning Memorandum on Some Thoughts About New Brands of Cigarettes for the Youth Market

URL: https://www.industrydocuments.ucsf.edu/docs/pspp0094 Author: Teague, Claude E. Jr. Document Date: 1973 February 02 Type: memo

Pages: 12

ID: pspp0094

TID: pny62d00

Collection: Joe Camel Collection

Mentioned: R.J. Reynolds Tobacco Company

Topic: Corporate Marketing Strategies, Targeting, Young Adults, Youth, New Products, Beliefs

Description: Draft memo/report suggesting new brands of cigarettes for the youth market. Memo expresses the feeling that if those 21 and under are smoking anyway they should be allowed to market to them and to do so R.J.R needs to develop new brands that are not already identified with the over 30 establishment market. Includes table: Effects Expected or Derived From Cigarette Smoking (Physical Effects, Psychological Effects for Pre-smoker, Learner, and smoker) which is then expanded on in the text of memo and product quality and product image concerns are also addressed.; Stamping and dark line obscure some information. For better copy see V001721-V001732

Availability: public; no restrictions Case: Mangini v. R.J. Reynolds Tobacco Company, Civil Case No. 939359 , Bates Number: 502987357-502987368 Bates Alternate: 502987357/7368; R.J.M027438/7449 Date Added UCSF: 2002 July 09 Date Added Industry: 1999 January 20

So, Bowen, Monsees, and eventually their angel investors, such as billionaire Nicholas Pritzker, were privy to a vast number of documents as the tobacco companies became saturated with lawsuits. Companies like R.J. Reynolds and Phillip Morris (now Altria), were legally forced to reveal their history, methods and additional private internal memos. Once these came into the public domain they were devoured by the founders of Juul, not as a cautionary tale, but rather as an actual "playbook." In other words, the effects of addiction were mostly disregarded in the pursuit of the model for marketing success. Human cost, in true sociopathic display, was dismissed, in order that the information could serve at the pleasure of the company. This information was in the form of documents that were studied by Juul, which was then acquired by Japan Tobacco International and funded by investors to the tune of $47 million. They learned how to manipulate nicotine to best develop an addictive product and examined tobacco companies' competitor products to see what had made them successful or not.

It was learned that R.J. Reynolds had known for decades that the product caused cancer but still struggled to produce a product and design that would secure "a larger segment of the youth market" *(LA Times)*. There were problems with palatability and not enough enjoyment or "kicks" (nicotine high) and episodes of people vomiting from inhaling too much; a problem later one of the former managers at Juul also reported in the "testing" phase. In fact, at Reynolds, the first generation of "nicotine salts" was patented in 1978. This proved to be the medium that could pack a punch of an excessive amount of nicotine with the least unpleasant side effects. All of this research and information was now in the public domain and available to Bowen and Monsees. See below:

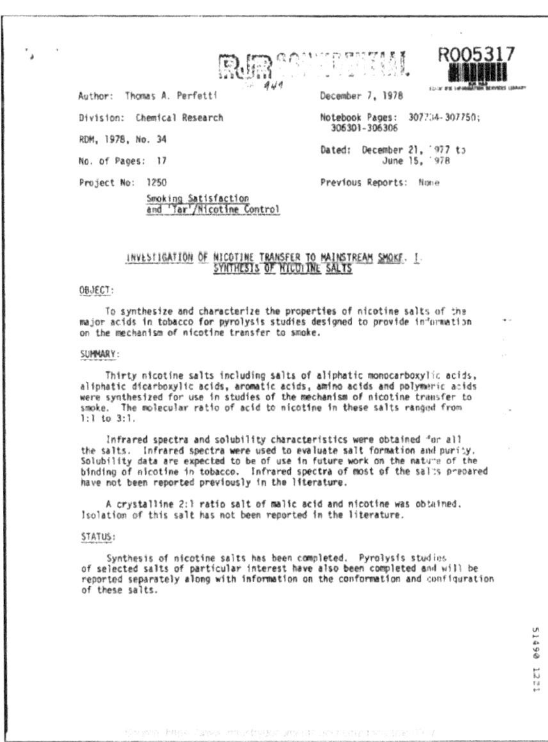

RJR CONFIDENTIAL
R005317

Author: Thomas A. Perfetti

Division: Chemical Research

RDM, 1978, No. 34

No. of Pages: 17

Project No: 1250

Smoking Satisfaction
and 'Tar'/Nicotine Control

December 7, 1978

Notebook Pages: 307734-307750;
306301-306306

Dated: December 21, 1977 to
June 15, 1978

Previous Reports: None

INVESTIGATION OF NICOTINE TRANSFER TO MAINSTREAM SMOKE. I.
SYNTHESIS OF NICOTINE SALTS

OBJECT:

To synthesize and characterize the properties of nicotine salts of the major acids in tobacco for pyrolysis studies designed to provide information on the mechanism of nicotine transfer to smoke.

SUMMARY:

Thirty nicotine salts including salts of aliphatic monocarboxylic acids, aliphatic dicarboxylic acids, aromatic acids, amino acids and polymeric acids were synthesized for use in studies of the mechanism of nicotine transfer to smoke. The molecular ratio of acid to nicotine in these salts ranged from 1:1 to 3:1.

Infrared spectra and solubility characteristics were obtained for all the salts. Infrared spectra were used to evaluate salt formation and purity. Solubility data are expected to be of use in future work on the nature of the binding of nicotine in tobacco. Infrared spectra of most of the salts prepared have not been reported previously in the literature.

A crystalline 2:1 ratio salt of malic acid and nicotine was obtained. Isolation of this salt has not been reported in the literature.

STATUS:

Synthesis of nicotine salts has been completed. Pyrolysis studies of selected salts of particular interest have also been completed and will be reported separately along with information on the conformation and configuration of these salts.

"Truth Initiative is America's largest nonprofit public health organization committed to making tobacco use a thing of the past." Earlier this year, CEO and President Robin Koval released the following statement:

Statement of Robin Koval, CEO and President, Truth Initiative® on the House Committee on Oversight and Reform's Subcommittee on Economic and Consumer Policy hearing, Examining Juul's role in the youth e-cigarette epidemic:

July 26, 2019

Congressional hearings about Juul's role in the youth e-cigarette epidemic proved, with the company's own testimony and documents, that Juul has become Big Tobacco 2.0. Committee members shared multiple exhibits that exposed how Juul's strategies and actions are straight from the tobacco industry's playbook. The startling evidence presented during the questioning of Juul co-founder and Chief Product Officer James Monsees, and Chief Administrative Officer Ashley Gould, indicates that:

- Juul misappropriated Stanford University's educational materials about youth prevention programs to the point of receiving a cease and desist from the school. Juul claimed they had no prior knowledge of how Big Tobacco used similar programs despite evidence indicating that they carefully studied the topic.

- Juul's logo so closely resembled Marlboro's logo design in the early days of the company that it resulted in a trademark infringement settlement with Philip Morris USA, whose parent company Altria ironically now owns a 35% stake in Juul.

- Juul programs targeted children as young as eight years old by funding summer camps, paying community and church groups to distribute their material, and targeting veterans' groups and other vulnerable populations.

- Juul continues to block and prevent Food and Drug Administration regulations, investing more than $1 million in lawyers and lobbying efforts in the last quarter alone. Meanwhile, Juul has failed to subject its products to the level of independent, clinical investigation needed to substantiate any claims of effective cessation, nor has the company applied to the FDA to be approved as a product to help smokers quit.

- At the same time as Juul admits to what they called marketing and education program "mistakes and missteps" in the U.S., they are implementing similar efforts in Canada, the United Kingdom and other parts of the world.

- Juul executives had trouble remembering many things under oath, including the fact that they had an entire department dedicated to social media influencer marketing clearly aimed at youth customers. James Monsees also seemed to contradict himself repeatedly as to whether or not Juul is in the cessation business.

- Despite Juul repeatedly claiming that it is not Big Tobacco, the company's actions and testimony tell a very different story. Through repeated misrepresentations, misremembrances and obfuscation, Juul showed itself to have studied the tone and tactics of the industry they claim to be trying to disrupt and to be taking them to a new level in what we can only characterize as Big Tobacco 2.0. The testimonies provided an abundance of new information and facts that we will share with young people through our **truth**® campaign to reveal how Juul is targeting and recruiting a new generation and putting their future health at risk.

As reported in Bloomberg, one more thing gave vaping an advantage. "The cigarette industry's record-setting $206 billion settlement in the 1990s severely curbed its ability to market to children and requires the companies to help cover state Medicaid costs for smoking-related illnesses. In 2009, Congress gave the FDA authority to regulate tobacco products to prevent kids and young adults from becoming addicts, which mostly meant banning flavored cigarettes and further restricting marketing. Companies would also have to get approval to introduce a new tobacco product. But at the time, the government didn't consider e-cigarettes a tobacco product.

The staff at Juul specifically studied the branding of Marlboro, one of the most successful brands ever, and deduced that their best chance for monetary success was to target a young demographic as Marlboro had. They learned that addiction that takes hold younger is likely to last a lifetime and also that individuals are not likely to start smoking after age twenty-five or twenty-six, so the optimal way to grow your business is to "get 'em while they're young."

In this way, it became apparent that it would be less profitable to switch adult smokers to vaping than it would be to market vaping to youth, and so the company's claims that early on their intent was altruistic and responsible were soon discredited as they abandoned the claims in all but lip service and as they set about engaging in all of the traditional youth marketing strategies. But there have been consequences.

We'll look into them later, as we follow a parallel process by first exploring how this crime was conceived, who conceived it, what circumstances either purposely or serendipitously enabled it to occur, how the victims were affected, who could have warned or helped the victims and ultimately, the consequences for the victims and perpetrators alike. For now, let's take a look at the findings below, widely reported across media outlets such as yahoo, nationalintrest.org, and on YouTube.

"In a major blow to the vaping industry, the American Medical Association has called for a ban on e-cigarettes and vaping products that the FDA doesn't deem tobacco cessation devices." Uh-oh. You can almost hear the corporate gasps. But that's nothing compared to the real "gasps" of increasingly more victims of vaping.

"As of November 20th, 42 people have died and more than 2000 have been sickened from vaping-related illnesses. By December these numbers had risen to 52 deaths and 2409 vaping-related hospitalizations. *The New York Times* reported last month on the youngest person to die from vaping, a 17-year-old boy from the Bronx."

CHAPTER 2

Anatomy of a Vape

In San Francisco, noted thoracic surgeon Dr. Wilson Tsai's practice has seen a steady growth in youth with pulmonary and tangential problems. He is often asked to speak and educate the public to the problem. Here are some excerpts from his interviews and discussions that illuminate and confirm the data:

Dr. Tsai:

I believe it's important to educate the public about what vaping is and what it does, because the rise in cases is epidemic; we've never seen anything like it. At the rudimentary level, vaping is a way to deliver a chemical that could be potentially mood-altering or have stimulating or depressive effects on the body. It's comprised of an energy source, a pen, which heats up a cartridge and creates a combustion. For example, when I light a match to a cigarette, combustion occurs. The tobacco is lit on fire and therefore the fumes from that are inhaled into the body. With the vaping pen, however, the pen is the heating mechanism not a combustion mechanism so the energy source that's delivered as a heat mechanism allows certain chemical reactions to occur. In order for that cartridge to dispense a vapor (the fumes), heat has to activate certain chemicals. They are required for combustion to occur. This process, along with the metals, can be carcinogenic and cause severe health risks. Other sorts of chemicals that have to do with enhancing flavors are also introduced and are extremely dangerous. One in particular, diacetyl, has been used in the past to flavor buttered popcorn. Years ago, there were factory workers who were having severe pulmonary complications from inhaling this flavor enhancer diacetyl, and they had tremendous lung damage and bleeding and so this became more commonly known as popcorn lung. The medical term for this disease is Bronchiolitis Obliterans. Think about that. Obliterating the bronchia. What that means is that the lung tissue has been damaged so badly that essentially there can no longer be an exchange of oxygen and carbon dioxide. At that point we'd call it end stage, destructive or terminal. Unfortunately, this very illness is making a comeback as we've learned in the story below from Canada. The *Canadian Medical Association Journal* confirms that an Ontario teen who was put on life support may be the first documented case of what's been known in the past as "popcorn lung," As mentioned, the diacetyl that provided the buttery or caramel-like flavoring, once heated is highly dangerous and when the 17-year-old ended up in a hospital emergency room he was initially diagnosed with pneumonia, due to his severe cough, shortness of breath and fever. But the antibiotics did not clear up the symptoms and he returned five days later in a worsened state. In addition to the breathing difficulties he was suffering fatigue and nausea. Upon questioning, the teen revealed that he'd been vaping heavily each day for the prior five months and that he'd bought his favorite flavored e-cigarette cartridges, green apple, cotton candy and dew mountain, online. He would often add THC to the liquid.

Despite supportive efforts and being put on a ventilator, the teen needed life-support saving interventions. One such treatment was ECMO. As described in www.thoracic.org and University of Iowa Health Care, ECMO, short for extracorporeal membrane oxygenation is a therapy that adds oxygen to a patient's blood and pumps it through their body like a heart.

It may seem unimportant to know the details of such a clinical intervention but consider the downplaying by the e-cig manufacturers coupled with the developmentally-appropriate and understandable "can't happen to me" feelings of teens. For that reason, these procedures shouldn't be sugarcoated. We owe it to the addicted youth and those enamored or soon to be enamored of vaping to describe the gravity of what can happen to a vaper and the treatment that, if they're lucky, may be needed to save their lives.

"In ECMO, also called ECLS, extracorporeal life support, the process takes place outside the body. It may be thought of as similar to a heart-lung machine used in heart surgery and can be used for longer periods of time. ECMO temporarily takes over the work of the heart and lungs so they can rest and heal.

ECMO is used when usual treatments are not working. ECMO does not cure heart or lung disease, it only provides time for the patient's heart or lungs to heal.

A surgeon places a plastic tube called a cannula into large veins or arteries. The blood vessels can be located in the chest, neck, or groin. The doctor may place different numbers of tubes depending on how ECMO is being used to help.

The ECMO pump pulls blood that has no oxygen attached from a vein and pushes it into the machine's artificial lung, or oxygenator. That's where carbon dioxide is removed from the blood and oxygen is added. There's a color change as the darker blood with no oxygen turns bright red when oxygen is attached to it. As the red blood leaves the oxygenator it is warmed before returning to the patient.

Because ECMO is also helping do the work of the patient's lungs, the ECMO team can lower the settings of the ventilator, allowing the lungs to rest and heal. Usually medications that have been used to help the heart and lungs function can be decreased while ECMO is at work."

Additionally, the Canadian teen required a tracheostomy. Here's how the Mayo Clinic describes that procedure. Tracheostomy is a hole that surgeons make through the front of the neck and into the windpipe (trachea). A tracheostomy tube is placed into the hole to keep it open for breathing. The term for the surgical procedure to create this opening is tracheotomy.

A tracheostomy provides an air passage to help you breathe when the usual route for breathing is somehow blocked or reduced. A tracheostomy is often needed when health problems require long-term use of a machine (ventilator) to help you breathe. In rare cases, an emergency tracheotomy is performed when the airway is suddenly blocked, such as after a traumatic injury to the face or neck.

When a tracheostomy is no longer needed, it's allowed to heal shut or is surgically closed. For some people, a tracheostomy is permanent.

This story has a happy ending. Though at one point his doctors were concerned that he wasn't going to make it, his condition slowly improved as he was also treated with high-dose steroids. His hospital stay lasted 47 days. And yet, despite his improvement, his airways remain severely obstructed. All signs point to the diagnosis of "popcorn lung" or its clinical name, bronchiolitis obliterans, but the medical staff felt it was too risky to take the extra biopsy needed to confirm. However, if the diagnosis is correct, he is likely to have some amount of chronic lung disease for the rest of his life.

While the personal stories, of which there continue to be so many, illuminate the "real life" situations, history is also important for context and it's helpful to understand a little bit of the history around smoking traditional cigarettes.

Years ago, the cigarette market was being heavily marketed to our soldiers. The campaign was that "you guys are at war, and you're going to kind of need this." They went after young guys that they knew had a whole life of addiction ahead of them. And many never quit. They just could never, ever quit. And at one time, before the warnings by the Surgeon General, there were even hearings in the Senate about tobacco and the lobby was so strong that the public was told that nicotine wasn't addictive!

Well, we all know it's addictive. And now, we have vaping, and they are wondering how we can convert young people who currently don't think it's cool to smoke. What an incredibly lucky fortune it would be to get them hooked on something else. And initially, the products were clunky and awkward and didn't sell well and didn't do the job of attracting young people enough. You see, it's almost like the mind of a drug dealer. How and where and who to target — where is your biggest market? So, when it came to the next generation, and especially to the makers of Juul, that was forefront in design and marketing. And young people? That's an annuity.

Sadly, our youth are also the most susceptible to addiction. They don't have full development in their brain, so introducing the drug makes them much more susceptible to addiction. Their prefrontal cortex hasn't been developed yet. And, talking about an annuity, the younger they are the faster and the more that they're getting addicted to it. That rate of return, every single year, is much more extended in the younger population, as described before with soldiers. Did you know that back in World War II our government was handing out packs of cigarettes to soldiers saying they should smoke them because it would keep them more alert?

And that's true because in essence, nicotine is a stimulant. And in low doses, nicotine stimulates your brain, it stimulates your heart, and so therefore, back then, it was touted as a favorable consequence of smoking, especially at war.

Now, when vaping first started, the products looked somewhat ridiculous, like those first Wall Street phones, like holding this big brick to your ear, and probably created a social stigma since it didn't look cool to have this thing that looked like a big banana that you're inhaling, that you're vaping from.

I think what Juul did as a marketing play was basically to make that design a lot sleeker, and in essence, it changed the social acceptance, and even probably elevated the social fashion to Juuling and to vaping. May times, now I see that vaping is equivalent to Juuling, because they've accomplished such a great control of the market in that sense. The kids use Juuling as a verb to approximate all vaping. And, you know, we joke around, that what they've done is really like taking a Honda Accord and making it look like a Lamborghini. But it's the same engine inside that Lamborghini, even if everyone wants to drive the shell to look like they're driving a Lamborghini. Unfortunately, it's just inhaling a drug, no matter which way you look at it, whether it be from the older clunky models, to these cartridges through a sleeker, USB-port-looking device. You are still introducing a certain drug, whether it be the nicotine, or the THC, into the body, to have that same desired effect, unfortunately.

And also, when they made the cartridges sleeker, there is a perception because they're so cute and tiny, they're not smoking that much.

And yet the opposite is true. In some cartridges, the concentration of nicotine can be equivalent to a pack of cigarettes, or some of them even a pack and a half of cigarettes. So, the fact that so much nicotine exists in one cartridge, and these youngsters are smoking one cartridge thinking that they're getting, for example, less delivery, they're really taking a super-amped concentration of a drug, and therefore are experiencing a much more heightened effect of that drug.

I think, at the same time, what happens with these cartridges is that the chemicals that are needed to allow the change from the liquid phase to the vaping or the gaseous phase, those chemicals, in addition to the nicotine or the THC, are extremely dangerous to a patient's health.

I often talk about diacetyl, but so much more can cause permanent lung damage. I worry about the metals in the devices, like mercury, nickel and tin. These are all heavy, metallic compounds that are required to facilitate the heating mechanism and the change from a liquid to a vapor substance.

This is important because many people aren't aware what happens to the cartridge, the casing, or things other than the chemicals. People often think they only have to worry about black market stuff and what you put *in* the cartridge. I would liken that to an alcoholic saying they don't have to worry about being an alcoholic or liver disease because they are drinking Johnny Walker instead of moonshine. When you look at it that way, it certainly casts a shadow on the "trustworthiness" of a high-end product like Juul.

See, the damage from vaping doesn't *only* have to do with what's inside. Think about the actual mechanism of vaping, what hot smoke does to your body as it goes down your esophagus and into your lungs. It goes everywhere. It goes into your heart, your stomach, and catches on so many of your vital organs.

Let me explain further:

First, there are **no** regulations right now regulating the amount of nicotine in a Juul cartridge, but regardless you still need an oil-based compound to be heated to form the vapors that will be inhaled. No matter what, when you place the cartridge in a vaping pen, the heat that's derived will cause the chemical reaction that transforms the liquid to gas and that process requires certain agents to be introduced. Just as we're now learning that with THC they had to put an oil-based Vitamin E compound in there and we know that oil inhalation can cause severe inflammation in the lung sometimes leading to pulmonary failure. In the past we heard the story of this when a small child inhaled a peanut. The oil from the peanuts causes this huge inflammatory reaction, which can cause these children, or these little babies, to be on a ventilator, while you're waiting for the lungs to heal from the inflammation caused by peanut oil.

So, once you know the anatomy of the vaping product, you learn that you heat it into the gas form and that gas goes down your trachea and into your lungs, and what happens because the lung is such a well-vascularizes organ in your body that the surface area to blood vessel exposure is extensive. Therefore, the mechanism of the effect of the drug is so much more potent. And so, the mechanism of the effect of the drug is so much more. And that's unfortunately seen as so favorable among young people. Instant gratification; the effects are immediate. You feel it more because you're not ingesting it. If you ingested it and it went through your stomach it would have to be processed through the body.

For example, marijuana edibles take a much longer time to feel, but with inhalation, the drug meets that blood vessel barrier within the lung and is distributed to cause systemic effects. There is massive oxygenation and then a vascularization of the lung. This can be felt in your brain, your heart, your lungs of course, and so forth. That is why people can get instant ventilation on ventilators. In the same way, you can have the reverse effect. One minute you are a healthy teenager and within hours you could be on a ventilator from vaping. This isn't something that happens over time and has a long causation like cigarette smoking or asbestos; this happens fast. Many of these young patients we're seeing have otherwise healthy lifestyles or are athletes. And primarily it has to do, as I said, with the chemical process of promoting combustion with the synthetic compounds in these cartridges.

I can't stress enough that it doesn't matter where you get it, whether it's on the streets of New York City or San Francisco or at a 7-Eleven or a grocery store or on the street. The minute that heated liquid goes into your mouth it's chaos for your body. I would like everyone to see the internal visual; because on the outside it can seem very glamorous, but on the inside it's basically like lighting your body on fire. Unfortunately, our young people are not being exposed to the warnings of the damage as much as they're being exposed to the "coolness factor"; it's even been said that the name Juul is a compound of **Jewel** and **Cool** (remember the cigarette brand Kool?) and what it really could be an anagram for is **Just Understand It's Undoing your Lungs**!! That's the advertising I'd like to see as the use by our young population becomes more and more widespread.

You see, when these kids have damage it can be seizures or strokes or cardiac events. This isn't likely to create small events, but serious catastrophic events. One thing I'd say is to err on the side of caution and with any symptoms, get kids to the emergency room as soon as possible. There are so many complications that can occur, depending on how frequently or excessively a patient uses and what the duration may be. We are seeing a set of patients with more chronic issues such as shortness of breath, persistent cough, many of the same symptoms we already attribute to cigarette smokers. At the same time, like the teen from Canada, we are starting to see the potentially terminal effects of vaping as these extremely healthy high school players end up on ventilators from excess vaping. There has been a huge spike in so many complications.

In addition to the pulmonary issues there is the serious issue of seizures and erratic heart rhythms. When the heart rhythm deteriorates, they need immediate medical attention and I should mention that hopefully insurance issues should not preclude someone from going to a facility immediately as no ER will turn away a patient in acute distress. But additionally, understand that even if the presenting problem is alleviated, patients and especially kids who've gotten to this point are looking at serious lifestyle changes. Certainly, someone can get off a ventilator. But if you have a cardiac event or a lung problem or lung cancer, this can affect you for the rest of your life. Just as there is a full spectrum of complications there is a full spectrum of ramifications. Some may even be looking at lung transplantation. And one of the inhibiting factors there is the limited availability. It's not like there are available lungs all over the place. They are scarce. In fact, a 17-year-old from Michigan has the distinction as being the first to receive a double lung transplant linked to vaping. The story has appeared in all the major media outlets including *The New York Times,* NBC news, *USA Today* and Bloomberg, among others.

Here, from *The Boston Globe:*

"DETROIT — A Michigan teenager was the recipient of what could be the first double lung transplant on a person whose lungs were severely damaged from vaping, health officials said Tuesday.

Doctors at Henry Ford Hospital in Detroit described to reporters Tuesday the procedure that saved the 17-year-old's life and pleaded for the public to understand the dangers of vaping.

The teen was admitted in early September to a Detroit-area hospital with what appeared to be pneumonia. He was transferred to Children's Hospital of Michigan in Detroit and taken Oct. 3 to Henry Ford Hospital where the transplant was performed Oct. 15. The double lung transplant is believed to be the first performed on a patient due to vaping.

Doctors found an "enormous amount of inflammation and scarring" on the teen's lungs, said Dr. Hassan Nemeh, surgical director of thoracic organ transplant at Henry Ford. "This is an evil I haven't faced before. The damage that these vapes do to people's lungs is irreversible. Please think of that — and tell your children to think of that."

Health officials declined to release the teen's name and said he is expected to recover. They also did not specify what the teen vaped or how long he vaped.

"We asked Henry Ford doctors to share that the horrific life-threatening effects of vaping are very real!" his family said in a statement released by the hospital. "Our family could never have imagined being at the center of the largest adolescent public health crisis to face our country in decades."

"Within a very short period of time, our lives have been forever changed. He has gone from the typical life of a perfectly healthy sixteen-year-old athlete — attending high school, hanging out with friends, sailing and playing video games — to waking up intubated and with two new lungs, facing a long and painful recovery process as he struggles to regain his strength and mobility, which has been severely impacted."

The boy had his 17th birthday after initially being admitted to the hospital.

Later in this book we'll look at exactly what happened, a story and message his parents have decided to make public on his GoFundMe page.

As mentioned, but should be mentioned daily, more than two thousand Americans who vape have gotten sick, many of them teenagers and young adults, and more than sixty people have died.

The Centers for Disease Control and Prevention announced a breakthrough into the cause of a vaping illness outbreak, identifying the chemical compound vitamin E acetate as a "very strong culprit" after finding it in fluid taken from the lungs of 29 patients. Vitamin E acetate previously was found in liquid from electronic cigarettes and other vaping devices used by many who got sick and only recently has been used as a vaping fluid thickener.

Many who got sick said they had vaped liquids that contain THC, the high-inducing part of marijuana, with many saying they received them from friends or bought them on the black market.

E-cigarettes and other vaping devices heat a liquid into an inhalable vapor. Most products contained nicotine, but THC vaping has been growing more common.

Henry Ford doctors did not say what the lung transplant recipient vaped. They did say that he was critically ill when he arrived at Henry Ford where he was placed Oct. 8 on an organ transplant waiting list. His lung damage due to vaping was so severe and he was so close to death that the teen immediately was placed at the top of the transplant waiting list, they said.

The double lung transplant of a teenager is an example of an extreme case, though Dr. Tsai suspects that despite being the first, his surgery and ordeal won't be the last. Here is another example from one of Dr. Tsai's patients, and the kind of case that he and his colleagues are seeing more and more frequently.

CARLY'S STORY

Carly, age 22, was brought to my office by her parents complaining of throat pain. Carly had been vaping, specifically with Juul, for approximately eight months. In her own words, with some extrapolation for content and coherency, here's what happened:

CARLY:

When I...I first tried it, it was probably two years ago, but I didn't start to vape two years ago. It probably was an eight-month period of my life from when I first started actually doing it. The first time I tried it, I absolutely hated it. I could not handle it. It did not rest well with me. I already have weak lungs. I have asthma to begin with and I just coughed up a storm, a huge coughing fit that lasted about five minutes. And I was like, "This isn't for me. I don't...I don't even like nicotine. I don't...I was just gonna give it a try, cause what's all the fuss about?" And so, I guess maybe six months later, it really got big. Like, more so than just a couple roommates doing it every once in a while. Everywhere you turned, people were doing it in class, on the street, even not just a Juul, just huge vape clouds on campus, everywhere. [Laughs.]

Also, I'm not sure if it was for fun, at least not for me, maybe for a lot of people it was more for studying. To be honest, I wondered why it wasn't working for me and also I don't really even like cigarettes, I've never smoked them. I don't even like the nicotine, it made feel kind of anxious and jittery and I didn't like that feeling but I think maybe it was like a subconscious addiction that I thought I just wanted to do it. In my opinion I think eventually it was easier for me to stop because I wasn't already a smoker and the people who are and then switch to vaping? It's not as easy for them to quit vaping.

I think it started off being the cooler thing to do. People always would say, "Oh you smell like cigarettes" or whatever. So, it started off like, very glamorous. But recently, I have seen some observable shift. Nothing too substantial but people are starting to say, like, "That's gross. Juuling is gross. Do you know what that does to you?"

For me, I think it just started, one day, when one of my friends was like, "I found this. I already have one. Do you want it? You don't have one so I might as well offer it up." And I tried and I thought...I, I... same thing happened, coughing, couldn't handle it. It felt terrible. It was painful. I thought, "Well, maybe this is just how it is...'cause I don't do it a lot. Maybe I'll just keep trying it and, like, it'll work for me, and then I'll see what...why everyone loves this so much." Um, and before you know it, like, probably a day into it, it just became...it was...like, my lungs got used to that feeling. Um, and that's when the addiction just started."

DR. TSAI:

I think what concerns me most is probably not the fact that she felt like her lungs were accommodated to it. I think what really concerns me more is the fact that, you know, in a day she got addicted to this. And so, I think that really lends to the danger of how one single cartridge of these vaping devices can have as much nicotine as an entire pack, or a pack and a half, of cigarettes. And you see that with someone who's younger, you know, the exposure to nicotine, and poor effects, because the prefrontal cortex isn't developed until you're 25 years of age, or more. Addiction compromises that part of your brain and it's the portion of your brain that's responsible for emotions and resistance to addiction, and because of that, in our younger population, the addiction potential is so much higher for them.

The second thing to recognize is that, especially in females, there's a trend that we know that females are more susceptible to nicotine exposure, nicotine addiction, as well as being more difficult for them to basically come off of nicotine as well. Studies have suggested that, potentially, there may be a difference between gender addiction and the difficulty to stop in the female population. But, again, it's very concerning to think that in one day she's addicted to vaping.

CARLY:

Well, I knew what the purpose of the…of the Juul was, is to get that nicotine high without smoking a cigarette. And so, the first couple times I tried it, I was so distracted by how my body was rejecting it and the coughing that I didn"t even want to continue. But then I was like, "Well, I didn't feel anything. I might as well keep trying." And so, that's.. I guess that's…I kind of tried it until I felt, like, "Oh, I see. Like, I get it now."

"Um, and then I think it, it just took off from there."

DR.TSAI:

And another statement I think is really important is how children (youth) are not saying it but they do want to achieve that nicotine high without smoking. And I think that's probably what these corporations have been very effective at, is trying to convince patients, and society that vaping is not smoking. So you've heard, you know, basically a lot of these, youngsters and young adults are saying that they're not smoking. But, unfortunately, the whole mechanism of smoking is inhaling a gaseous product to deliver the drug. So, unfortunately, you know, that message has been lost because, I think, the marketing supersedes the reality of what's really going on.

CARLY:

I would go to the gas station with 20 bucks and I would probably…if my gas light was on [laughs], I'd put five in the tank and then spend the other 15 on the Juul pods at the gas station. But then the next day at work I'd get…you know, I'd just get enough gas to get by for that day and then I'd get the pods just because, you know, it's easy just to go up to the register and just…. It was that easy. And the truth is, back then, I would rather buy pods than food, gas, or cosmetics.

Now we all see stuff on the news every day now and new cases of death and kids on ventilators but it also seems like no one thinks it's going to happen to them. We don't know anyone that it's personally happened to. And there are arguments from people, counter arguments about the stories in the news that we don't know exactly what the illnesses and deaths are from. They talk about pre-existing conditions and if that's what you want to hear, especially because you're addicted and don't want to give it up, that's what you'll hear. Even though we see it that thousands of kids have issues, and hear from the parents, and see the filed lawsuits and see it on social media now, there's this false perception that people who've smoked cigarettes for twenty years are fine so of course I'm going to be fine since I've only vaped for eight months.

I know they don't realize everything they're inhaling and all these different factors that play into it. And like how technology really has changed something as, not simple, but something like tobacco into having so many more chemicals to keep it preserved and keep it like, vaporizable and like, whatever they have to do. And so, you know, comparing it to cigarettes, they think they have all this time to quit and I don't think it really resonates with anyone until it's going to be too late. I'm directly surrounded with people who aren't taking it as seriously because in my community there hasn't been a sensational case.

However, I did hear yesterday that Boulder, Colorado actually raised the prices or something and the age requirements for buying Juuls from 18 to 21. So, there is some awareness but it's baby steps. Also, I heard they banned all flavored liquids. But the thing is now a lot of people are just into the menthol and saying that's even better. And I feel like that's what differentiates the people that are truly addicted to the nicotine aspect of it from people like me that are just kind of like...the mint did taste good. It didn't make my breath smell bad. It was accessible and it was easy but you know, the fact that they only sell flavors that kind of taste like what you're trying to avoid, would probably turn me away from it altogether because I don't think that I genuinely like it myself.

I also want to, it's really everywhere, all over school. I could probably walk one block from campus and pass three stores where I could get them. You can get them at 7-Eleven, they have the widest variety, but there are also smoke shops on my college campus. I would even get messages from some of these vape shops that "We're having a huge Juul sale!" And the prices dropped before they passed the age restriction to, I would say to a third of the price of a Juul starter pack, so I guess it was to make it more affordable to students.

They would check my student ID; I will say that. Since I started in college, it was pretty much that everyone was already of age. But I do have friends whose younger siblings tried to get it. I mean, if you want to get it...it's kind of like alcohol. If you want to get it, you'll find someone who's going to get it for you.

So, I don't know. The age restriction is definitely a step in the right direction but you know, I'd be lying if I said if I hadn't bought alcohol for the nineteen-year-olds around me at school.

Technically you're also not allowed to vape just like you're not allowed to smoke in places. I've had bartenders come up to me before, me and my friends, and say, "You do that one more time, you're going to get kicked out of here."

And I know to do it on an airplane is like a $200,000 fine and it's especially dangerous to do on an airplane. But people do it. They go into the airplane bathrooms and even with the smoke detector in there they vape. And yeah, I know at restaurants, too, because I was doing it; I used to take a break from work and go in the bathroom because I could hide there.

DR TSAI:

Shortly I will share information and advice for parents, but I think it's important to discuss what young people like Carly would recommend for parents, to help them keep their children from vaping. And also to applaud you, Carly, for stopping. And if you could share a bit about how you were able to do that, how you became motivated and determined?

CARLY:

I would say first, that there just needs to be more light shone on how it directly is related to all of these health issues. I think, like I said, people are not really...that's not really what they want to hear. And so, when they see things like this come up, you know, they try and blame it on something else. So we need to dispel those myths.

But I think I would really just say, to parents, like, you've got to stand your ground. Tell kids to just stay away from it. You know, save your money. Spend your money on other things. And I mean, it's really hard to get into someone's head to make them really not want it.

But I'd really just suggest they urge to them how important it is to realize, like what this is doing to people. How it's... it's literally taking over lifestyles in certain situations. Like I said, when you're compromising your grocery list so that you can afford cartridges, it really all comes down to a lifestyle change and you know, if you...I hate to say it but if you really, you know, if you need to chew the Nicorette gum or whatever, do whatever you can but like, I just think that like, the inhalation of that vapor; what that's doing to people's lungs is happening more discreetly and rapidly as it ever has before.

For me, with my weak lungs, I had symptoms right away, bad symptoms. So, I would lay down at night just after a whole day of vaping and feel or think about all of the negative ways it was or could be affecting me. My hair did get thinner. My skin looked more tired, and it just formed this big negative picture that became empowering to change.

I also had some friends who quit with me. We just threw them away. Threw them out. Physically threw them away and you know, like, decided that we were going to do things that put us in the right direction. And we kind of started looking at it, I guess, from a more mature perspective than…just a college culture of it being the cool thing to do, like, "Oh, I'm so addicted to the Juul." It's like, embarrassing to say that but at the same time people will think that's what college is all about, that culture.

So, I guess I would say that taking the mature road and getting a couple friends to like, join you on the way and then sitting back and noticing how your life is improving positively works; it becomes more positive reinforcement to stay away from it.

DR TSAI:

It's an excellent point that we now know that there are many conditions that occur as a result of vaping that haven't yet come fully to light, such as skin issues, hair loss, autoimmune illnesses; many major inflammatory responses to toxins.

It seems that Carly has talked about all the necessary steps to essentially recover from addiction. You know, it's funny, because when you tell someone that they're addicted to the Juul they have a strange reaction to the word. They see addiction as something that has happened to someone who has hit rock bottom and lost all their finances from it, all their relationships, and so on and so forth. But quite honestly, that's not what addiction is about. It exists on so many different levels. She also figured out a way to use peer pressure positively, rather than be led down a negative path.

CARLY:

Well, I would like to pay it forward. One of the things that I noticed that kind of drove me to stop was when I was doing it at work and some of my older…not old, just a couple years older than me co-workers would just be like, "Oh, I just think that's disgusting." And just hearing that word associated with it after all this glamour and all this pizazz or whatever is supposed to be the connotation for the Juul had an impact. Hearing someone kind of talk down to me but not even to me felt awful. Knowing she thought it was disgusting bothered me.

So, I guess maybe…not talk down to people but, but urge them. Put words like that in direct connotation with vaping and that lifestyle.

And especially talk about this false perception that, "Oh, like, so and so's been smoking for 20 years. They're fine. I'm gonna be fine. I've only been vaping for eight months."

Make sure they know they're not realizing the difference in what they're inhaling and all those different factors that play into it and, like, how technology really has changed something as...not simple, but something like tobacco into adding so many more chemicals to keep it preserved and keep it, like, vaporizable and, like, whatever they have to do. And so, you know, in comparing it to cigarettes, they think they have all this time to quit, and I don't think it really resonates with anyone until it's gonna be too late.

To read more about the dangers of vaping and to listen to the podcast with Dr. Tsai and Carly, visit www.HIVE80.com, the fastest growing social media community for health and wellness, or follow the link below:

https://hive80.com/hives/hive-vibe/forum/topic/the-hive80-podcast-dr-tsai/

Dr. Tsai is only one of many medical experts to be alarmed. Consider the following: A Reuters Investigation looked at the way that addiction can set in quickly among young vapers. Susanne Tanski, a pediatrician and former chair of the tobacco consortium at the American Academy of Pediatrics, said she and colleagues are observing first-time Juul users becoming addicted within two months, compared to two years or more for a smoker to become dependent on cigarettes.

And, according to a study last year by scientists at the Roswell Park Comprehensive Cancer Center and Stony Brook University in New York, they found that the levels of a nicotine indicator in the urine of young regular users of Juul or similar e-cigarettes was nearly 60% higher than that of regular cigarette smokers of the same age. Which leads one to wonder whether it's possible or even likely that young vapers may be ingesting more nicotine.

Researchers at Harvard Medical School and Massachusetts General Hospital surveyed more than 1,600 high school students in the Boston area and found that 58% of those who had ever tried Juul or similar high-nicotine devices continued to use them, compared to just 17% of teenagers who had ever tried cigarettes.

"The person who is becoming addicted to cigarettes has to be more determined; they almost have to want to become a smoker," said Dr. Jonathan Winickoff, a pediatrician at Mass General Hospital for Children in Boston, who was involved in the survey. "With Juul, you get trapped much more easily. There's nothing about it that's telling your body that it's harmful."

Couple this with the latest information regarding Juul, specifically, and it's no wonder we're dealing with an addiction epidemic. On January 6th, 2020, Channel KPIX in San Francisco reported that "rodents that had been exposed to Juul test **eight times higher** for nicotine concentration than a competing e-cigarette and 5 times higher than a traditional cigarette." Think about the adolescent experimenting for the first time with no baseline for nicotine consumption. While an adult switching from traditional cigarettes may physically intuit when they've "had enough," what chance does the first-time teenager have against the powerful addictive concentration in Juul? One might ask, "How would they NOT become addicted?"

This paints Juul as reprehensible as Big Tobacco and no differently than the drug dealer on the corner. More about this latest research and the devastating physical and behavioral effects of Juul can be found at : https://sanfrancisco.cbslocal.com/2020/01/06/ucsf-juul-nicotine-vs-cigarettes-e-cigs-study/.

Across the board, the experts that weigh in on the dangers of Juul and vaping consistently warn that there hasn't been enough time to test the long-term effects of the products and process. It's no surprise, then, that the more time that goes by, the more the damaging results come to light. Consider the two findings that have also been uncovered in January of 2020:

First, a Harvard research team has discovered a toxin in Juul and other e-cigarettes that can cause severe inflammation in the airways when airborne; in other words, inhaled. This microbial toxin called glucan, contributes to lung inflammation and can create asthma, emphysema, chronic bronchitis and Chronic Obstructive Pulmonary Disease or COPD. Even more astounding is the way that all of these conditions can occur in otherwise healthy people. But scarier still is the finding that glucan was found in 80% of all e-cigarettes, including Juul, and that the greatest concentrations of glucan are occurring in menthol and tobacco flavorings, the very two that Juul has NOT pulled off the shelves and continues to manufacture. Yahoo lifestyle, when citing the Harvard study states what a great number of medical professionals have feared, that "the e-cigarette product may not be the harmless smoking cessation device that Americans were promised."

The second revelation comes from the site, www.hive80.com, which released the findings of a study that ties vaping to increased chances of stroke. The study states the vapers are twice as likely to suffer a stroke as traditional smokers and three times as likely as those who don't smoke at all. This study comes out of the neurology department at the University of Kentucky and is not surprising to most in the pulmonary community who have already recognized the extreme risk that comes with vaping or smoking any substance in terms of physical damage and addiction.

As the medical experts note, due to the development in young people's brains which can continue at least up to age 25, early addiction sabotages the normal and healthy progression of processes in the prefrontal cortex such as executive function, decision-making, acquiring knowledge, emotional regulation and rationale. And no one is sure just what the long-term effects of nicotine might be. Surprisingly, most long-term studies have not focused specifically on nicotine, even in traditional cigarette smoking because the other known toxins took center stage. Newer studies do suggest that much harm to teenagers' brains is likely.

Instead of following the developmental path that leads to growth and full function, the neuropathways are interrupted by the substance.

Counselors at addiction treatment centers know that when it comes to addiction, chemicals that occur normally in the brain such as serotonin, dopamine, melatonin and even adrenaline, are said to "turn off." In other words, the brain takes a little vacation because the depressant or stimulant "has got that covered." Think about some real-life situations.

- A teen with poor decision-making may take risks or make poor choices. It doesn't take much to imagine all the ways this might cause harm or death.

- A young adult who used to being stimulated or "high" suffers from depression when the substance is removed. It's common to hear teens in early "recovery," before the serotonin returns, remark that "everything is boring" and they are tired all the time.

- A young person is firing so "hot" with adrenaline that their anxiety is off the charts. Think about the "fight or flight" function of the amygdala, the brain's anxiety regulation center. What happens when it is over-stimulated? Patients with panic disorder and generalized anxiety disorder report feeling that they are in "flight" all the time. School-refusal and school-avoidance are at an all-time high.

Though many brain functions can return over time, this is a slow process that may take years, and the younger the patient is when first addicted, the harder it may be to regain normal function. Some studies show that stimulants create an almost insatiable need in some youngsters. This can lead to more and more dangerous substance use in later years. High schools and colleges have gotten the message and are sharing the warnings.

For instance, At the University of Texas MD Anderson Cancer Center, the community service homepage states the following:

A Smoking Prevention Interactive Experience (ASPIRE) is a free, bilingual, online curriculum, fully aligned with National Education Standards, as well as with 21st Century Skills, that helps middle and high school teens learn to be tobacco free while explaining the dangers of tobacco and nicotine use.

The program is evidence-based and tackles the full range of traditional and emerging products such as e-cigs, hookah, Juul and synthetic marijuana. Assessments are imbedded and gauge users' knowledge before and after exposure to the curriculum.

- Students can earn a certificate of completion upon finishing the program.
- Click on "Student Log In" to begin.
- Teachers/Administrators can see students' progress by logging in to the Admin site.
- Healthcare providers can refer teen patients to this engaging tobacco/nicotine resource.
- Anyone can see what ASPIRE offers to fit their needs by clicking on "ASPIRE Select."
- User support is provided.

Within the site are further warnings on the harmful effects of vaping:

The risks of vaping

Researchers do know that e-cigarette aerosol contains toxic chemicals like those found in glue and paint. What's less clear is if the amounts are high enough to cause diseases like cancer.

"The biggest problem is that we don't know exactly what goes into all the flavorings, and there are thousands of them," says Robinson. Experts say it could take 20 years to know the long-term health effects of vaporizing.

But there are some clear dangers to e-cigarettes, particularly when it comes to nicotine.

Nicotine is addictive. In fact, it's one of the most addictive substances available. An addiction to nicotine can lead e-cigarette users, especially kids, to escalate to regular cigarettes.

"The fear is that these young people who would never have tried cigarettes are now getting dependent on nicotine at the most impressionable time," Robinson says.

Nicotine is harmful. This is particularly true for young, developing brains. Nicotine use can stunt an adolescent's ability to learn and affect their behavior. It lowers their ability to resist addiction, leading to more nicotine use. Nicotine also worsens conditions like depression and anxiety.

If you have asthma, e-cigarette aerosol can irritate your throat and lungs.

If you're a smoker, vaping could support your habit, not break it. Instead of transitioning from cigarettes to e-cigarettes, some smokers end up using both.

"There's no evidence that people can switch and stay switched, some people go on to dual use," Robinson says. "They may cut back on cigarettes but they use e-cigarettes to get nicotine in areas where smoking is banned."

This increases their nicotine addiction instead of lessening it, he says.

Nicotine patches, nicotine gum and other smoking cessation products are designed to help smokers wean off nicotine. Unlike e-cigarettes, they are proven to work.

The liquids and devices can be dangerous. e-cigarettes have been known to explode and the fluid is poisonous if it comes into contact with eyes or skin, or if you accidentally or deliberately drink it.

Robinson says the reasons for avoiding Juuls and e-cigarettes are compelling.

"If you're not already dependent on nicotine, why take the risk of becoming addicted and damaging your health?" he says. "If you are dependent on nicotine, you are much better off using safe cessation tools that are proven to be effective to curb your cravings and get off tobacco products."

Finally, if you are a smoker, any non-tobacco based nicotine product is better, he says. But try prescription or over the counter forms before e-cigarettes.

Concerns are high across the board. Google almost any state, or any high school or college website in the country and you will find a cautionary tale. Here is a sample, with multiple excerpts from www.edweek.org:

NEW JERSEY

9 hospitalized with mystery illness in N.J. after vaping. Here's what we know.

By Kelly Heyboer, NJ Advance Media for NJ.com

"New Jersey health officials are on the hunt for more cases of young people suffering from lung ailments — including coughing, shortness of breath and fatigue — after nine people in North Jersey were hospitalized after using vaping products.

The New Jersey Department of Health issued a statewide health alert Friday asking health care providers and local health departments to report any cases of unexplained lung problems in people who use e-cigarettes and other vaping products."

NORTH CAROLINA

As reports accumulated of people stricken with lung disease after they used e-cigarettes, important clues emerged from a local emergency department.

By Sarah Ovaska-Few

A North Carolina hospital offered some of the first clues into what's been an ongoing medical mystery, the vaping-related lung injuries that have killed 18 people in the country to date and sent more than a thousand to hospitals with serious injuries.

Officials with the Centers for Disease Control and Prevention announced the new death count Thursday afternoon and continued to strongly urge people to avoid using any vaping or e-cigarette devices given the current dangers and unknown nature of the current health crisis.

"I wish we had more answers," said Anne Schuchat, CDC's principal deputy director. "This is a critical issue."

Doctors at the WakeMed Raleigh campus saw three relatively young adults come in within a week of each other this summer, all struggling to breathe and with no other obvious signs of what could be causing their distress, said Kevin Davidson, one of the critical care pulmonologists at WakeMed, in an interview with N.C. Health News."

OHIO

Columbus — Three second graders in one Ohio school district were caught with a vape pen.

In another district, a superintendent said he has a student with a $150-per-week vaping habit. Those stories are just the tip of the iceberg. Vaping in Ohio schools has become a pervasive and costly issue. Students caught doing it are disciplined and miss class time while districts are now spending thousands of dollars on vape detectors to combat the problem.

Across the state, the number of vaping incidents in Ohio schools has skyrocketed by more than 700 percent since 2016, according to a months-long investigation by WBNS-TV's investigative unit, 10 Investigates.

The reporting was done in partnership with our TEGNA sister stations, WTOL in Toledo and WKYC in Cleveland.

Ohio schools are not required to track vaping incidents, meaning until now, there has been no readily-available or centralized data to track the problem.

10 Investigates, along with reporters at WTOL and WKYC, reached out to more than 600 school districts across the state.

Four-hundred-fifty school districts got back to us and 353 gave us specific information on vaping.

What we found uncovered an alarming trend: vaping incidents in Ohio schools have skyrocketed from 773 two years ago to more 6400 incidents last school year — a 732 percent increase.

THE UNIVERSITY OF VIRGINIA

"Nicotine will actually alter the structure of a developing brain, and we have no idea what that will do in the long run," said Robert Klesges, a professor at the

University of Virginia Cancer Center. "[A]ll the adverse health consequences that we know about in e-cigarettes are short-term health consequences, and it will be 30 to 40 years before we know how dangerous e-cigarettes are."

But many teens are not aware of the hazards of vaping. Sixty-six percent of teens believe their e-cigarettes contain just flavoring, according to the National Institute on Drug Abuse.

WISCONSIN

At Arrowhead Union High School in Hartland, Wis., about 27 miles from Milwaukee, administrators installed devices in the bathrooms over the summer that detect vaping and automatically send email alerts to the associate principal. And high school students trained in prevention education will be deployed to the middle schools to talk to younger students about the dangers of vaping, according to Principal Gregg Wieczorek.

"I would rather convince a kid to not start, than to ever have to convince them to stop," Wieczorek said.

COLORADO

The Boulder Valley School District in Boulder County, Colo., has moved from letting individual schools decide how to handle such incidents to developing a community-wide approach that now stresses prevention efforts, including education for students about the risks and how to make good decisions, and informational parent nights that feature the county's public health department, law enforcement, local doctors, and experts.

They are also working with local physicians to ask screening questions during regular check-ups. About 33 percent of Boulder Valley high school students vape.

The district is backing a series of measures before the Boulder City Council that would ban the sale of flavored nicotine and tobacco products, increase the minimum age to buy nicotine and tobacco products from 18 to 21, and push a voter-approved city sales tax on such products.

WASHINGTON

"It's been a challenge for us administratively in all of education, and it's a challenge in society," said J. Eric Diener, the principal of Eisenhower High School in Yakima, Wash., where tobacco or marijuana use more than doubled between 2017 and 2019 and the confiscation of illegal devices like vapes went from just four in the 2017-18 school year to 36 in 2018-19.

Experts agree that vaping is harmful to students' bodies and brains. There are toxic chemicals and metals in many e-cigarettes, and vaping can cause respiratory issues, and potentially cardiovascular problems, and even seizures. The nicotine itself is much more concentrated in e-cigarettes than traditional ones.

SOUTH CAROLINA

After hearing from principals that they need help dealing with "blatant" incidents of vaping, including an instance where students had videotaped themselves vaping on campus, the Horry County school district in South Carolina will have a mandatory three to five days out-of-school suspension for the first offense if they are found with e-cigarettes or smoking-related devices.

Tobacco violations in the district, which include using e-cigarettes, more than doubled over two academic years, jumping from 427 incidents in the 2017-18 school year to 1,030 in the one recently completed.

"They [principals] wanted more teeth" to the policy, "and a little bit more flexibility," said Lisa Bourcier, a district spokeswoman, who added that education and cessation have always been part of the district's response.

FLORIDA

Last month, Florida's Hillsborough school district and the sheriff's office launched a public service campaign called "Put Down The Pen" to urge students to stop vaping. It highlights some of the consequences they could face if they are caught.

In addition to suspension, students face a possible felony charge if the liquid in the vape pen includes a banned substance like tetrahydrocannabinol (THC), an ingredient in cannabis.

"We want to educate them so that all of the students know the discipline they may face in school, but, also if it rises to the level, how it can affect their futures if law enforcement gets involved," Hillsborough spokeswoman Tanya Arja said.

As of this writing, Reuters cites the CDC report of 2,758 cases of severe lung illnesses tied to vaping in recent months in the United States. Nowhere is it more apparent than in the state of California, which has issued the following from CDPH, its Department of Public Health.

"The California Department of Public Health (CDPH) urges everyone to refrain from vaping, no matter the substance or source, until current investigations are complete. Since June 2019, CDPH has received reports that 169 people in California who have a history of vaping were hospitalized for severe breathing problems and lung damage, and four people have died. Across the U.S., there are over 2,290 reports of lung damage associated with vaping across 49 states, the District of Columbia, Puerto Rico and the U.S. Virgin Islands, and more reports are coming in nearly every day."

CDPH, along with other states, the Centers for Disease Control and Prevention (CDC), the U.S. Food and Drug Administration (FDA), local health departments, and healthcare providers are working hard to investigate what is in the vape materials that is making people sick.

Although CDPH regulates manufacturers of cannabis vaping products to ensure they are as safe as possible for those who choose to vape, CDPH warns that individuals put themselves at risk any time they inhale a foreign substance into their lungs. The risk of vaping now includes death. CDC continues to warn that any tobacco product use, including e-cigarettes, is unsafe, especially for youth, pregnant, and breastfeeding women.

Sudden lung damage from vaping is a new health problem.

We are learning from this investigation that lung damage can happen very suddenly to people who vape, including people who have not been vaping for a long time, and young, healthy people who do not have lung disease or other health problems. This is different from most other health issues caused by vaping and smoking, which happen over a long time and can be worse in people who have other medical conditions. Additionally, most patients do not have a recent history of smoking regular cigarettes, suggesting these lung issues are exclusively related to vaping. Many types of vape products may be causing the lung damage from vaping.

Almost all people with lung damage from vaping say that they vaped or "dabbed" the cannabis products THC and CBD in cartridges, waxes, oils, and other forms. Some people report vaping only nicotine. Many people report vaping a combination of both nicotine and cannabis products. The investigation is still in process, but the one thing that people with the lung illness have in common is a history of vaping.

County health departments are contacting the people who had lung damage from vaping to find out which products they used, where they purchased the products, and to collect their vape products to test for harmful ingredients.

The government does not ensure the safety of vaping devices through regulation. In California, licensed cannabis retailers are required to sell products obtained from a licensed cannabis manufacturer that have been tested by a licensed laboratory. Cannabis products sold by licensed sources are tested for a variety of chemicals, pesticides, microbial impurities, and heavy metals. Illegal cannabis dispensaries sell unregulated and untested cannabis products and absolutely should not be used.

People are hospitalized with breathing problems and other symptoms.

People with lung damage from vaping typically have symptoms that start a few days to a few weeks before they go see a doctor. All people hospitalized developed some type of breathing problems, but many people also have other symptoms. The symptoms reported by those who have gotten sick are:

- Breathing symptoms: trouble catching their breath, coughing, chest pain.

- Gastrointestinal symptoms: nausea, vomiting, diarrhea, abdominal pain.

- Non-specific symptoms: feeling tired, fever, weight loss.

These symptoms are very similar to having a lung infection like pneumonia or bronchitis, so it can be hard to tell if the symptoms are from an infection or vaping the first time someone sees the doctor. There is no test that a doctor can do to know that breathing problems are from vaping right away. Laboratory blood tests and an x-ray or CT scan of the lungs may be necessary.

People with vaping-related lung disease are usually admitted to the hospital because of their breathing problems.

- Teenagers and young adults make up almost half of the people hospitalized with breathing problems from vaping in California.

- 30% of people hospitalized in California had to be treated with a mechanical ventilator, or "life support," in the intensive care unit (ICU).

Be aware that your child's respiratory issues could be related to vaping.

Parents should be aware that numerous cases involve children under age 18. Parents in particular should be aware that e-cigarettes and vaping devices are available in more than 15,000 flavors that may be attractive to children, such as mango, bubble gum, unicorn poop, mint. The secondhand aerosol typically smells sweet so it can be hard to detect. Be aware of the symptoms in case your middle or high school child develops symptoms, and seek medical attention.

No one knows yet why this lung damage is happening from vaping.

There are many different possible ingredients added to cannabis and nicotine to make the cartridges, waxes, and oils used for vaping. Multiple people who were diagnosed with lung damage from vaping say that they received the cannabis products from unlicensed smoke shops or individuals. Vape products sold by unlicensed retailers are not tested and can contain harmful ingredients. We do not know yet if all of the people in the country with this illness use the same vape products, or if the products were contaminated with the same substance.

The long-term effects of vaping are still unknown, but these short-term effects are alarming.

Recommendations for the public

1. CDPH urges everyone to quit vaping altogether, no matter the substance or source. For those who continue, you are urged to avoid buying any vaping products on the street and never modify a store-bought vape product.

2. If you, or your child, have vaped at all in the past few months and are having new problems with breathing or other symptoms, you should seek medical care immediately and tell your healthcare provider about your history of vaping.

3. If you decide to stop vaping, do not replace vaping with smoking combustible cigarettes. Ask your doctor for FDA-approved quitting treatments.

CHAPTER 3

Befriending and Grooming the Victim

A veritable fruit salad of available flavors of Juul cigarettes flooded the market in June of 2015. Cucumber, Crème Brule, Blueberry and flavors that caused one middle schooler to remark, "tastes like donuts and cereal!" were purportedly intended to make the experience pleasant. Juul founders continued to contend that their products were created to help adult smokers switch from tobacco cigarettes to a safer method of enjoying "the magic and luxury of smoking," yet this statement proved faulty and dangerous on two fronts.

First, key components that were uncovered in the tobacco documents, some referenced earlier, showed that scientists examined how to get users over the initial barriers for a young person to start smoking. These included the aversive and harsh results of nicotine ingestion that are hard to take: coughing, nausea, dizziness. At this point, Juul had a choice. If, in fact, they were attempting to attract smokers and help them switch to a less harmful product, there was no need to make the experience less harsh than smoking. One could argue that the opposite would hold true and a fruity or pleasant experience would be a barrier to smokers switching. Additionally, they could have reduced the amount of the addictive substance, nicotine, in their product. But they did not. Instead, they devised a delivery system whereby a combination of benzoic acid and nicotine in the form of a salt delivers the nicotine in a way that practically eliminates any harshness and allows for the delivery of more nicotine than any other e-cigarette with no harshness. Let's explore an acronym for how Juul marketed to our youth. I call it **FADS**. Flavor, Addiction, Design, and Social.

First, let's talk more about the **F** in Fads, **FLAVORS**. They are endless. In addition to those already mentioned, the flavors smack more of Baskin Robbins or Dylan's Candy Bar than "an adult product." Think gummy bear, cotton candy, peanut butter cup, cookies 'n cream, pop rocks, chocolate, wild berry, watermelon, lemonade and menthol. There is literally a website called Flavors Hook Kids (www.flavorshookkids.org) which is powered by Tobacco Free California. The governor of the state has issued an executive order and released a statement on the site that says "With mysterious lung illnesses and deaths on the rise, we have to educate our kids and do everything we can to tackle this crisis."

The National Institutes of Health claim that four out of five kids who vape use flavors and that kids 15-17 are more likely to use Juul than older groups. Almost all studies suggest that the flavors draw kids into smoking/vaping in a way that cigarettes haven't in years; first because they think it's cool and safe, but mainly, because of the fruity and minty flavors. A government study found that 81 percent of kids who have ever used tobacco products started with a flavored product, including 81 percent who have ever tried e-cigarettes and 65 percent who have ever tried cigars. 81.5 percent of youth e-cigarette users cite flavors as a major reason for their current use of non-cigarette tobacco products.

As it turns out, years ago, the big tobacco companies did try to hook kids with flavors. Finally, legislation was passed under The Tobacco Control Act in 2009, which gave authority to the FDA over tobacco products, and flavors other than menthol were prohibited. Unfortunately, the FDA only had this authority over tobacco and no other products such as e-cigarettes. Because the flavors are luring kids into vaping, an entire culture is changing. The campaign to keep kids from smoking worked and the number of teen smokers dropped dramatically in recent decades. All of that is being eradicated by vaping and especially flavored vaping and the other "advantages" of a Juul pen. Think about this: The percentage of cigarette use among kids of high school age has declined by 70 PERCENT since 1997, from 36.4 percent to a record-low 10.8 percent in 2015 while the number of underage vapers has skyrocketed.

Consider the following from the CDC:

• Tobacco product use is started and established primarily during adolescence.

• Nearly 9 out of 10 cigarette smokers first try cigarette smoking by age 18, and 98% first try smoking by age 26.

- Each day in the U.S. about 2,000 youth under 18 years of age smoke their first cigarette and more than 300 youth under 18 years of age become daily cigarette smokers.

- Flavorings in tobacco products can make them more appealing to youth.

- In 2018, 67% of high school students and 49% of middle school students who used tobacco products in the past 30 days reported using a flavored tobacco product during that time.

- Recent increases in the use of e-cigarettes are driving increases in tobacco product use among youth.

- The number of middle and high school students using e-cigarettes rose from 3.6 million in 2018 to 5.3 million in 2019—a difference of about 1.7 million youth.

Parents are often stymied. A story on www.fastcompany.com describes how one mother fought a losing battle despite trying desperately to keep her kids from vaping. She was so concerned and confused that she even thought of offering to buy them a vaping system that did not deliver nicotine. She then learned about what she calls "Juul's dirty tactics," such as posturing the device as innocuous, and packaging it in a way that parents would be unaware of what the product was, and while making multiple flavors, none were offered with non-nicotine options.

Of course, she heard the standard arguments from her kids, like "everyone's doing it." We know that oftentimes that's a teenage tactic for whatever they'd like to be doing and oftentimes it's false. But as many parents are learning, when it comes to Juul, the statement is not as suspect as you might think. Parents nationwide are shocked to learn that, as one parent calls it, not only has Juul been marketing aggressively to teens in multiple venues and ways, but that there has been "an all-out assault on the habits of my son's generation" by Juul since its launch in 2015.

Let's talk about the **A** in **FADS**, **ADDICTION**, and about nicotine.

Pharmacologist James Pauly, a specialist in nicotine, notes that Juul delivers more nicotine than other e-cigarettes, and that the salts also may reduce the harshness, making it easier for new smokers, such as teenagers, to consume more nicotine than they are aware of. How much nicotine? Estimates are that each Juul pod contains the approximate equivalent of 1-1.5 packs of cigarettes, or 2-300 puffs. So, if a user goes through one Juul pod a day, that is the nicotine equivalent of smoking at least a pack of cigarettes a day.

Nicotine is thought to be as addictive and tough to quit as heroin. Remember, that cigarette smoking causes a slow deterioration over many years and vape pens deliver much more of a deadly punch. But what exactly does nicotine do to a teen's body? We know it's a stimulant, as Dr. Tsai has explained, but let's not sugarcoat; nicotine is a neurotoxin some call Brain Poison. In a free newsletter specifically distributed to students, www.sciencenewsforstudents.org, the following is stated:

"Nicotine acts like a key to unlock special receptor molecules on the outside of cells in the brain, including those in the prefrontal cortex. Nicotine causes these cells to release signaling molecules, such as dopamine. These chemical signals travel across a gap between nerve cells (called a synapse). When they reach the neighboring nerve cell, they release their 'message.' And it gives users a feel-good high."

But after repeated exposure to nicotine, those brain cells can change. The effect of these changes is to reduce the body's ability to release its own, natural pleasure-giving chemicals.

Meanwhile, the brains of teens who smoke or vape may create more receptors to handle the flood of nicotine they have come to expect. As the number of receptors increases, teens will need more nicotine to get the same high. That makes nicotine users seek hit after hit. In teens, this can provoke side effects. For instance, it can make it hard for them to stay focused. It might also trigger bouts of depression or anxiety. Some of the negative effects of nicotine on the young brain will fade with time — if exposure ends. Others, however, may persist. For instance, brain scientists at VU University Amsterdam found that exposing adolescent rats to nicotine increased their impulsive behavior. It made them a bit more reckless than usual. It also made it harder for them to focus their attention — even later, as adults.

No one is sure that the same thing happens in humans, but that's the concern. Exposing the developing adolescent brain to nicotine "could lead to a high risk of lifelong addiction," says Garry Sigman, head of adolescent medicine at the Loyola University Chicago Stritch School of Medicine in Maywood, Illinois.

When we think about nicotine addiction, we tend to focus on the physical and the ensuing emotional problems. But let's look at adolescence itself, a tumultuous time many of us remember with angst and confusion and/or many of us see our own children going through. Phrases like "brain development" seem clinical and in some ways at arm's length. An adolescent struggling with the normal, expected changes in hormones and neuropathways who then becomes additionally taxed with addiction, is going to have consequences. They may isolate more, socialize less, act out differently or aggressively, experience mood swings or sleep deprivation, among so many other differences. This may play out in school, at home and at work. The adolescent who is addicted is at risk for erratic behaviors, feelings and actions. Just think about how that plays out for all of us.

Dr. Tsai points out that most of these young people are at the beginning of their lives. Perhaps they want to go to college, graduate school, become a professional or just simply succeed. If you don't have your health it makes it much harder to accomplish your goals and the rate of failure is almost certain to go up with the rate of disability. The world is competitive and these young people are stacking the deck against themselves through using these products. They will be competing with those who never vaped, who are not compromised, and everything will be harder. Also, the combination of being high on anything and largely connected to the world through electronics can make for its own combustible concoction.

What we can learn from Dr. Tsai and so many of his colleagues in the medical field is that there may be many tangential issues waiting in the wings, so much fallout we don't even realize yet, fallout that will be the result of this vaping epidemic. Adolescence and young adulthood is a time to learn about relationship-building, distress tolerance, emotional regulation, and self-esteem. All of these processes are interrupted or altered when someone is developing while high.

Let's also not ignore that a vaping pen is a drug delivery system and young people dealing with peer pressure have a tremendous amount of exposure to the cultural legitimacy of marijuana. Now that pot is legal in many states so its use is on the rise. And we know that these pens have become a convenient way to deliver pot, sometimes without any smoke or odor. We know that many new vaping atrocities are due to the combinations of THC and other chemicals like Vitamin E required for combustion. But also, it's important not to minimize the pot!

As Dr. Tsai says, marijuana is not a safe drug! Now that we've made it easier to bring marijuana to this demographic in a handy, colorful, barely visible gadget, we also have to consider the consequences of long term marijuana use begun early, sometimes in the pre-teen years. Let me tell you about a client of Dr. Tsai's we'll call Mike.

Mike is a 40-something with metastatic lung cancer. That means it's not just confined to his lungs but has spread throughout his body. The most common places lung cancer spreads are the liver, the bones and the brain. When he was asked if he smoked cigarettes he denied it. Eventually he was asked about marijuana. Mike revealed that he'd been smoking quite a bit for 15-20 years. He had no idea that the marijuana smoking was the cause of his cancer and had always believed it to be safe. He was shocked. Yet his reaction is not uncommon. Most young people think that marijuana is a safe drug, but any drug, used excessively or abusively, is dangerous.

We cannot overlook what doctors like Dr. Tsai are trying to tell us: Their patients are getting younger and younger. Typically, a pulmonary patient was age 50, 60 or older, now many more high school students are coming in with pulmonary complications and the one thing that is almost always identified is their vaping.

You see, students gather around things that look "cool" or "grownup," and even a little rebellious. Individuating that way can be seen as a normal part of development, just as kids may be well-behaved at school but terrors at home. This is natural, to test emotions and behaviors "where it's safe." Years ago, kids would gather in the school bathroom to smoke cigarettes. Simply put, vaping is causing massive and extensive pulmonary damage unseen in smokers of the past.

Often, Dr. Tsai has advice for parents. The world will glamorize vaping, but you must discuss the dangers with them. And not only with scare tactics. Kids are smart. Even middle-schoolers today understand and scour the internet about subjects that interest them. If you educate them to the scientific dangers and even to the way that the business of vaping, the marketing and such, targets kids for profit, they may hear it. Kids can understand how big business appeals to them with flavors like cherry Kool-Aid and bubble gum and how those who want to make money will disregard the health of the public. They will understand when you talk to them about "fine print" and how no one is mentioning that the product contains nicotine let alone how much! They will understand chemical reactions and "lighting your insides on fire." Sometimes parents want immediate confirmation that their kids have heard them but we know that if the message is consistent if will have an effect whether they give you the satisfaction of knowing if it did or not.

There are things parents can look for; nose bleeds, exhaustion, kids that lock up their backpacks or their clothing or when these same items or their rooms smell like the fruity flavors we've mentioned. Obviously you want to stay involved and engaged with your children and know what they are doing, but if you actually do know that your child is vaping, you have to accept that there may be an addiction going on and not deny it. Kids will deny and bargain or minimize and minimize it next to cigarette smoking and if you accept that attitude you're not going to be of help to them. When your child is not acting right or seems bothered or upset or there are changes in personality or energy or anxiety or mood swings, you have to investigate. Especially heightened irritability, lethargy and poor sleep. I suggest open discussion, not punitive measures. Ask the questions and encourage honesty so that you can then have an educating discussion about how vaping truly is drug abuse and be heard rather than ignored. This is especially important because of the climate we live in today we where we medicate children with an assortment of pills for everything from ADHD to anxiety.

I'm not saying that pharmacological treatment is bad, only that if the cause is nicotine addiction and we treat anxiety with meds, we'd be missing the problem. We call that the poly-pharma root where we are prescribing all sorts of symptomatic medications and missing the root cause. Another thing you may uncover if the teen is vaping marijuana is that then THC needs to be dealt with as well. So as always, open communication is the key.

Finally, make sure to reiterate that there really is no safe smoking product. Vaping is not safer than cigarettes, cigars or a pipe. Marijuana is not safer than nicotine. It's all smoking. It's all drugs. Just as you'd never tell an alcoholic to keep drinking but switch from scotch to beer, you don't tell a smoker to switch to vaping; different dangers but always dangerous. "Vaping is smoking, vaping is using drugs, vaping is dangerous" and I think those are three messages we really have to give our society.

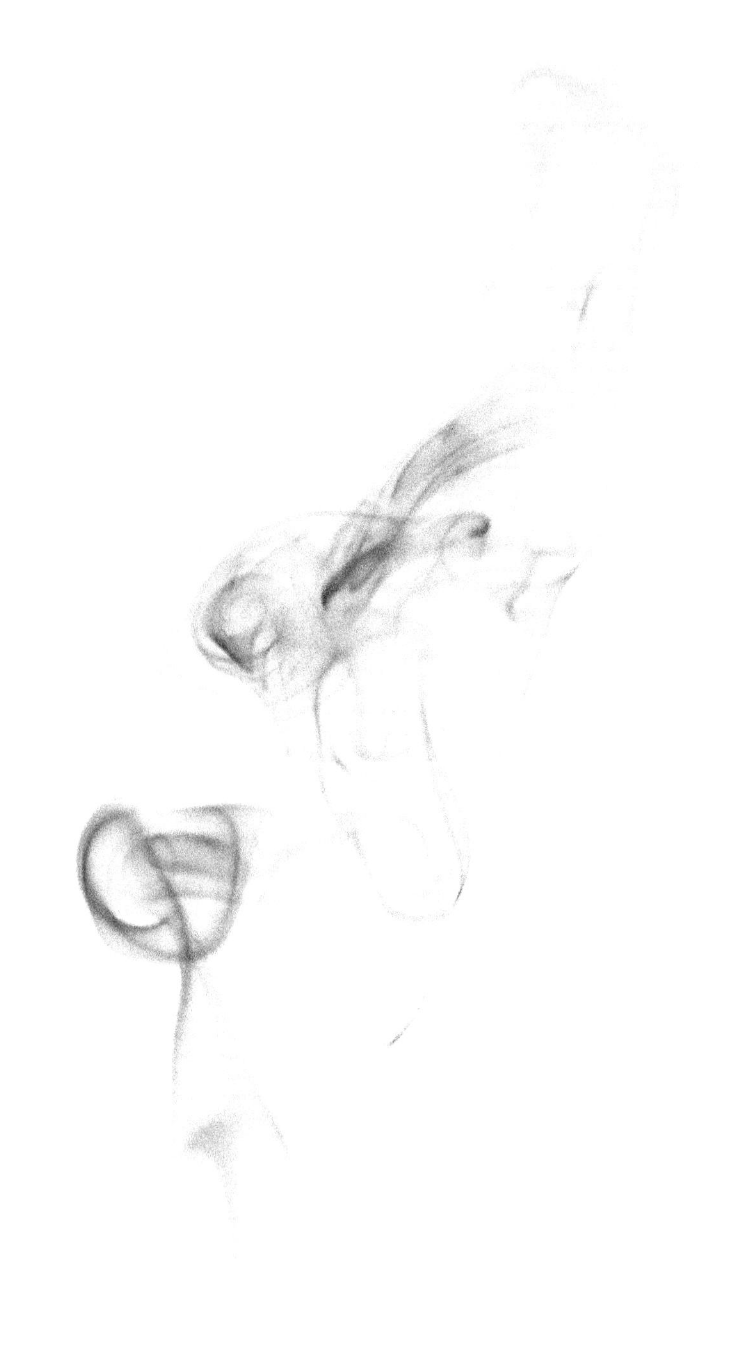

CHAPTER 4

Vape, Pillage and Burn

Next, a look at the **D** in **FADS, DESIGN**. Not only were the Juul pods *Flavored* and super-charged with nicotine to promote *Addiction,* but the e-cigarette was *Designed* to be sleek and techie and advertised as such. In fact, a Juul product could be hidden in the palm of a hand, or a sleeve, or a bra. It looked like it could be charged in any USB port, ultra-cool and minimalist and deceptively like a flash drive so that parents would not be suspicious, and it was small enough to be easily hidden. Women will remember the way that pocketbooks began to include an inside pocket for cell phones some years ago. In the same way, some companies, not associated with Juul, even began to incorporate a Juul hiding pocket in their products (www.vaprwear.com) and kids discovered they could easily fit the product inside a Sharpie marker.

From ABC13 Houston a video on YouTube shows how high school kids are hiding their vape pens in an ordinary watch. https://www.youtube.com/watch?v=w4I IqXlgUmoQ

Also on YouTube is a post called "Vaping 101, Best Places to Hide Your Vape/Juul #2." They suggest pencil cases, an old DVD box, in a pair of shoes, and the most ingenious, the pocket of a tie. This post has almost 30,000 views.

"Where to Hide Your Vape" has 294, 000 subscribers and Part 1 of 5, posted in March of 2019, has over 700,000 views on YouTube: The young man who posts continually uses a Juul pen throughout the video. He says he's using a fake Juul pod, the watermelon flavor. It's clear that this poster is high. From the laconic drawl opening of a drawn out "What's up," to his frustration with his Juul not lighting ("Fuck Juul"), it's painful to think that underage kids might be watching this video and thinking it's cool to Juul. He does begin the video by saying that he doesn't endorse vaping by minors, and yet...check out the content. His advice includes eyeglass cases, DVD boxes (but make sure it's one that nobody in the family watches!), a deodorant stick (take out the stick, and fill the hole with your vape), cutting a seam in your mattress or box spring (parents will just love that one), or, finally, cut out pages in a book, or in your teddy bear. In terms of the last one, he says he doesn't have a teddy bear because he's a "grown-ass man." We can, of course, assume that his disclaimer about speaking to minors is disclaimed.

https://www.youtube.com/watch?v=BlMYyEUi1io

A short internet search on How to Hide a Juul reveals a list of places and ways, such as:

- How to hide a Juul in school

- How to hide a Juul from your parents

- How to hide a Juul on a plane

- How to hide a Juul going through a metal detector

- How to hide a Juul in a Sharpie

- How to hide a Juul in luggage

And most frightening, "How to hide a Juul from TSA and airport security."

Take a look at this thread on reddit.com regarding hiding a Juul, last year:

How to Properly Bring Juul on a Plane?

First off, I am legal age in my state to buy Juul pods, but my parents don't know I Juul. I am taking a flight with them soon and I was wondering what the most hassle-free way to get my Juul with pods through security is. Thanks.

The answers to the thread ran the gamut from a theme of "man up" to "no worries" as the TSA security check seems to let the pens and pods go through easily whether in a backpack, wallet, or the security bins. Not sure which is scarier, based on that information; that the items are easily concealed or allowed. As it turns out, vapes, pens, e-cigarettes and pods are allowed in your carry-on but not in your checked suitcase. In fact, they are only allowed in the main aircraft cabin. Really? After all, there have been so many scary stories of late regarding vape pens blowing up.

In fact, back in 2017 an e-cigarette started "smoldering" on a Sky West flight to Los Angeles and in September of that year a backpack with four vaping batteries caught fire during boarding. In February of 2019 a Delta flight to Houston from New York was canceled due to a vape pen emitting smoke in a passenger's carry-on bag prior to take off and Southwest employees pulled a smoking suitcase out of the cargo hold in San Diego; both the plane and other luggage were damaged. This statement is reported from The Washington Post:

"An FAA advisory group said last year that the agency's guidance for flight crews in fighting fires caused by electronic devices is "inadequate and outdated." It said better training is needed to manage threats from burning batteries, including potentially toxic and flammable gases and smoke that could obscure pilots' vision.

"'So far, we've been lucky nothing's happened,' said Charles Leocha, president of the advocacy group Travelers United. 'I just don't think the FAA has caught up with the threat.'"

From early 2017 to present, as reported in multiple media outlets including *The New York Times,* CNN and CBS News, we've heard stories across the nation about these devices blowing up and not just harming the vaper but causing explosions of varying degrees. The Daily Beast reports on the increase in visits to emergency rooms and trauma centers due to exploding e-cigarettes. What can be extrapolated from the article, in addition to the facts, is that this "safe" product not only has dangerous implications from its substances, but from the external device itself and the battery that often charges it. Injuries are horrific: stories of painful shrapnel destroying tissue and bone, jaws broken, being doused in blood and burning plastic. Other damage can result in broken teeth, face fractures, and large chunks of skin being literally ripped away.

FEMA's U.S. Fire Administration reported that between 2009 and 2016, serious incidents from e-cigarettes exploding jumped from 15, to 38, to 98 in 2016 and these were just the cases that were reported; true casualties could be much higher. A 38-year-old Florida man was reportedly the first person to actually die from an exploding e-cigarette in 2018. In some instances, a person can suffer a "blast injury," and have an artery severed. This happened to a 24-year-old in Texas. He, too, died.

And in New York, a worker in Grand Central Terminal was severely burned when an e-cigarette exploded in his pocket. Witness Byron Gonzalez reported that "Seconds after the 'sparking and sizzling' began, we witnessed his pant leg explode. Out of nowhere a huge explosion came from one of his pockets and it just shot at us." Apparently vaping isn't just threatening to the user. While the workers at Grand Central were unharmed, it's reported that an accident in Utah caused first and second degree burns to a mother in her car when her vape pen exploded. Not only was she hurt, but the blast caused the copper coil to fly into her son's car seat. Generally, burning causes the most damage, it's reported, and the most pain. E-cigs that explode in the mouth can cause third-degree burns that require extensive scraping and grafting and damage can include nerve loss while the chemicals that explode may cause second-degree burns.

The FDA has taken some steps to keep consumers safe, offering public workshops, guidelines, safety tips and regulations of batteries. Juul is one of the companies that insist they, too, are taking steps. A Juul spokesperson told The Daily Beast, "Juul Labs takes product safety incredibly seriously, which is why each device is inspected multiple times before it leaves our manufacturing facilities. Our devices are specifically designed with multiple protections, while charging and in use, and have undergone rigorous testing in a wide variety of scenarios."

Vuse, a company owned by tobacco titan R.J. Reynolds that issued a voluntary recall of 2.6 million vape pen units in April 2018, said they had since improved "process," "quality controls," and "the charger accessory," and that the company "take[s] pride in providing our consumers with tobacco and vapor products of the highest quality."

A representative from the nonprofit advocacy group American Vaping Association emphasized that these events are extremely rare — and that many of the e-cigarettes that have exploded have been mods.

"Users of devices like Juul or virtually any product with an internal battery have nothing to fear from this story," AVA President Gregory Conley told The Daily Beast via email. "However, for those consumers wishing to use more advanced products that require batteries to be removed for recharging, learning and practicing battery safety is a must."

But the authors of the *NEJM* report disagree. "Although these explosions were previously thought to be isolated events," the authors wrote, "the injuries among our 15 patients add to growing evidence that e-cigarettes are a public safety concern."

One of the premier lawyers taking on Juul is Brooks Cutter of Cutter Law (https://cutterlaw.com). He claims:

"One of the main concerns regarding e-cigarettes is that the batteries can either on their own or while inside the e-cigarette explode, causing serious burn injuries to users.

Consumers whose e-cigarettes use lithium-ion batteries could be at risk of having the battery explode and cause injuries. If the user is engaged in other activities at the time the battery explodes such as driving a vehicle the injuries could be devastating.

Among the circumstances that can lead to a lithium-ion battery exploding are contact with other metal objects, extreme temperatures (either high or low temperature), overcharging the battery, or using a poorly-designed charger."

It should be noted that Juul devices do not appear to carry the same risk of explosion because while they do have lithium-ion batteries, they are not the kind that have been exploding (18650s) and need to be taken in and out. Juul batteries are designed to remain permanently in place.

"The manufacturer of Juul specifically worked with the battery manufacturer to design a battery. They have overcharge protection," said George Kerchner, president of the Rechargeable Battery Associations, PRBA, in an interview with NBC News.

A recent Netflix documentary once again describes the way that Juul took a page from Marlboro advertising, advertising that is now prohibited for tobacco, and duplicated the same sort of message. Juul showed its product being used by young adult models that could pass for 15-year-olds. The visually bright colors and scenes of sexually attractive, fun-loving gatherings, as well as celebrities, were practically irresistible to emerging adolescents wanting to fit in. The messages promote relaxation, independence, travel and success: a teenager's holy grail.

And these images were plastered in all the right places: a pop-up store in The Hamptons, a billboard in Times Square, an ad in *Vice Magazine.*

An interesting report published on www.Vox.com describes the white paper created by a team from Stanford, called Stanford Research, into the "Impact of Tobacco Advertising." Led by Stanford professor Robert Jackler, the team studied Juul's marketing campaign between 2015 and 2018. They used multiple tools, studied thousands of Instagram posts, emails, and ads, as well as the company's own Facebook, Twitter and Instagram accounts, many, many emails to consumers, and even used a program called Internet Archive Wayback Machine to uncover ads and strategies that had since been discontinued. When all was said and done they published this finding:

"Juul's marketing was patently youth-oriented.

Their stated goal was to try and uncover the impact of appeal to young people. They created a system, rating and coding for several topics, including youth appeal, humor, pop culture, use of memes, cartoon imagery, covert use of the product, Juul tricks, and Juul as an alternative to smoking."

They noted that Juul's product launches also occurred at sampling events in major U.S. cities. Their product was freely handed out at movie and music events and the study deduced that the aim of the free samples was to create exponential use of Juul products by young people and young influencers. Asking them to accept the products, try the products, and spread the word.

It's also hard to overstate the appeal of the Juul design. The Juul is so small that students report being able to "rip a Juul" during a high school class, either by making a hole in their sleeve and resting their head on their hand, or clipping it to the front of their shirt and doing the same. And the warning labels? Initially non-existent, although due to recent pressure they have been added.

As described in one YouTube video on "Why Altria Bought 35% of Juul," the product is considered the "Apple" of design, and in terms of visuals "your Juul would fit nicely in with your Apple and Tesla."

https://www.youtube.com/watch?v=G0zTOlCrT54

So, let's be clear: The Juul is not your father's Marlboro Man. And the only horse in sight is the hoarse cough of the user. As we continue to explore just how appealing the design and the ability to conceal has been to kids, here are some horrific quotes from high school students that permeate the Netflix documentary and other articles:

"I thought it had only water vapor."

"70% of kids at my high school vape and like 95% have tried it."

"I hit it 40 times a day."

"I tried to quit but only made it a week or two."

"I guess one more time won't hurt."

"I've seen every type of kid vaping; athletes, theatre kids, brainiacs."

"I would never smoke real cigarettes."

"Sometimes I'm happy to wait a little longer between hits, 'cause then I get a bigger buzz."

"I get lightheaded when I vape."

"If I need to hide it when I'm vaping, I 'zero it in,' which means I keep it in a long time so no smoke or air comes out."

"Don't worry I'm not using an e-cigarette, I'm using Juul."

"When I run out of pods I get so upset and tired and irritable. I need it!"

"My allowance was small but I would spend all the money I had on pods."

"So. I spent like $1300 a year, I did the math."

"I just vape because I'm addicted. I really don't like it."

"I honestly don't think it's possible to quit in this [high school] environment because of how many there are around."

If vape is inevitable...relax and enjoy it??!!

Another design tactic of Juul, in particular, was not just bright colors but creative and artistic patterns. On Amazon and other sites, this product runs the gamut from looking like a high-tech tool to an ultra-glam cosmetic. Plus, not only did they highlight the pretty packaging but at the same time they did not list the nicotine or any of the other ingredients. That's changed now, likely because of public uproar, but think about the initiation. The same kids who wouldn't dare eat sushi from ShopRite were lining up to buy an unknown ingestible liquid from the convenience store. Today there are 22,000 brands of vaping products and thousands of flavors. And most kids still don't know what's in them. What's more, of the 7000-plus flavors of Juuls, not one has been studied to see if flavoring actually helps smokers quit.

There are proven safe ways to quit smoking. Though success statistics are not as overwhelmingly effective as one would like, the solution doesn't kill you. Smokers have a choice.

WEB MD lists 5 ways to quit smoking:

- Cold Turkey, which is the most tried and least successful.

- Behavioral Therapy, which involves exploring your triggers and making a plan to get through cravings.

- Nicotine Replacement Therapy, which includes nicotine gums, patches, inhalers, sprays and lozenges. Best used in combination with Behavioral Therapy.

- Medication, such as Bupropion and varenicline (Chantix) to help with cravings and withdrawal.

- Combination, a mix of several methods (but not two nicotine replacements at the same time) in a "cocktail" that works best for you.

Additionally, many sites such as www.quit.com offer programs, plans and information to help. Some sites, like www.smokingcessationformula.com offer free webinars and alternative methods for quitting. One wellness site on the east end of Long Island, N.Y. even offers laser treatments combined with acupuncture to help smokers stop. (www.laserforquitsmoking.com). And the American Society of Clinical Hypnosis website, www.asch.net, can help you find a certified clinical hypnotist in your area. While not personally endorsing any of these sites or methods, the message is clear. Smokers who want to quit have a myriad of safe options to try without vaping.

This brings to mind an old smoking cessation program called SMOKENDERS which has been financially revitalized and now exists online, though years ago it occurred in person (group support!) in seminar and meeting rooms formats. The program helped many smokers quit by addressing the addictive certainty of nicotine and its withdrawal symptoms as well as the behavioral component of habitual smoking. Today, therapists know this as an arm of Cognitive Behavioral Therapy or CBT. The program allowed smokers to slowly wean off the nicotine and tars in cigarettes over several weeks: The first four or six you could smoke, as long as you changed brands (interrupted familiarity) and each change was to a cigarette with less and less nicotine. There was a mindfulness component. Every cigarette was logged with a short note about why you wanted it and had it. No judgement, just a consciousness about the choice. Studies have shown that when it comes to any addiction, be it food, alcohol, or the "process" addictions like shoplifting, a log brings the behavior into consciousness and works to reboot the automatic nature of consuming or acting without thought.

Concurrently with nicotine reduction, in SMOKENDERS, behaviors also had to change; it was required that each week you eliminate smoking in a room you would usually smoke in, and that you change how you hold the cigarette as well. Again, each week you'd eliminate a room and some hand/fingers you'd typically use. Some smokers reported that by the end they were holding the cigarette between their left pinky and ring finger, smoking a cigarette that was "all air," and doing it in the downstairs pantry and they almost couldn't wait to stop smoking altogether. In other words, rather than making it EASY to smoke, the program made it uncomfortable and unpleasant and eventually more of a chore that just didn't feel worth it. This is the absolute antithesis of Juul, who did everything they could to make it comfortable to vape, who did everything they could to make teens unaware of what they were smoking.

In SMOKENDERS there were other mindfulness components. All cigarette butts had to be put out in a water jar and you had to look at them throughout the program; watch the water getting dirtier and blacker and smell. Also, there was a money jar; every time you spent your money on cigarettes you had to put an equal amount in the money jar so you could see over time how much you spent on your habit.

Finally, there were intellectual pieces that were at the core of CBT. In other words, change your thoughts, change your feelings, change your behaviors. One in particular was about what was happening to your body the minute you finished a cigarette. It addressed nicotine addiction by explaining that the minute you stopped ingesting the nicotine, the actual minute you put the cigarette out, the body would begin the cycle of craving it again and the desire would build. And it challenged the things you told yourself about your feelings. It challenged your "self-talk." Because smokers would and do often refer to certain cigarettes (first thing in the morning, after coffee, dinner, or sex) as "a great cigarette." They will say, "Man that was a great smoke."

But SMOKENDERS reframes that "great cigarette" as simply a relief from pain, relief from the pain of nicotine urging and need, and asks participants to think about a headache, which is pain, and ask themselves this question: If you had a headache, and took Excedrin, would you ever say, "Man that was a great aspirin!" See? Smokers, and now vapers, or JuulERS, have been duped. Once you're addicted, one more cigarette, one more puff, one more pod, no matter what flavor it is, is simply a relief from pain, the pain of nicotine addiction.

Now let's examine the final **S** in FADS, **Social.** Or more accurately, social media. And Juul was one of the first major e-cigarette brands to rely heavily on social media to market and promote its products

One study found that Juul's initial marketing expenditures in traditional channels were modest compared to competing brands, but that these advertising efforts have effectively reached youth and young adults.

The Surgeon General concluded that "e-cigarettes are marketed in a wide variety of channels that have broad reach among youth and young adults." The 2016 National Youth Tobacco Survey (NYTS) found that 78.2 percent of middle and high school students — 20.5 million youth — had been exposed to e-cigarette advertisements from at least one source and found that exposure to e-cigarette advertising is associated with current e-cigarette use among youth and that greater exposure to e-cigarette advertising is associated with higher odds of use.

In fact, in a recent CNBC article Rep. Raja Krishnamoorthi, chairman of the House panel that oversees consumer product investigations, says that e-cigarette maker Juul is breaking the law in advertising its nicotine pods as a safer alternative to traditional cigarettes and tool to help people quit smoking.

We need to think about how young people get their information. Think about how they connect to the world. Most educators and parents are concerned enough about the lack of "real connection" between young people today; so many are attached to their electronics, to their tablets, phones, and computers, and these false walls are built up by social media and kids forget that one post can cause a lifetime of pain. They also have difficulty with eye contact, conversation, and a host of other tech-related social fallout that has therapists seeing child anxiety in record numbers. But social ramifications aside, social media is the sandbox of today; it's where our kids feel out who they are and want to be and where they get messages about what's cool and what's not, misguided though those messages may be. Who do you think has more followers, socialite Kim Kardashian or Nobel scientist May-Britt Moser. Right.

Guess how many hashtags there are around Juul? Here's a sample:

#Juul, #Juulpods, #Juulnation, #Juulvapor, #Juulgang, #Juulnmemes, #Juuling, #Juultricks, #Juullife, #Juulcenteral, #Juuls, #Juulpod, #Juulskins, #Juulcompatible, #Juulcharger, #Juulvape, #Juultje, #Juulmango, #Juulstarterkit, #Juulmoment, #Juulfam,

Think a curious teen trying to fit in might possibly find a product or two?

To further understand the disregard for potential harm to young people, let's remember that Big Tobacco companies like R.J. Reynolds and Phillip Morris were subject to congressional hearings as far back as 1994 and to a fault, each representative, six to eight men, lied to Congress when they stated, "I don't believe that nicotine is addictive."

It's been reported that not only did they know they were lying but so did everyone else. And more, they knew that cigarette smoking was causing cancer and death and had for two decades.

And yet, the founders of Juul decided to glean whatever they could from these companies to create a blueprint for how to market and sell their product. What they didn't do was try to make it safer. Let's also take a look at some of the cautionary tales that began to emerge as early as 2015.

First, remember the Stanford study reported on Vox? They also concluded that what had the biggest impact on luring youth was not necessarily what they were saying about the product but how they got the word out in the media. Robert Jackler is quoted as saying:

"What Juul did that's different is it exploited social media, where American middle and high school kids live."

And while so much buzz has been on Juul's innovative mechanism and delivery system for that pleasant nicotine experience and taste, Jackler says about their use of social media, "That was their real innovation."

Juul also hired social media influencers with large followings and created the hashtags we mentioned before and cool campaigns about "vaporizing." Which showed young people much in the same way as YouTube videos showed tricks or jokes with their Juuls.

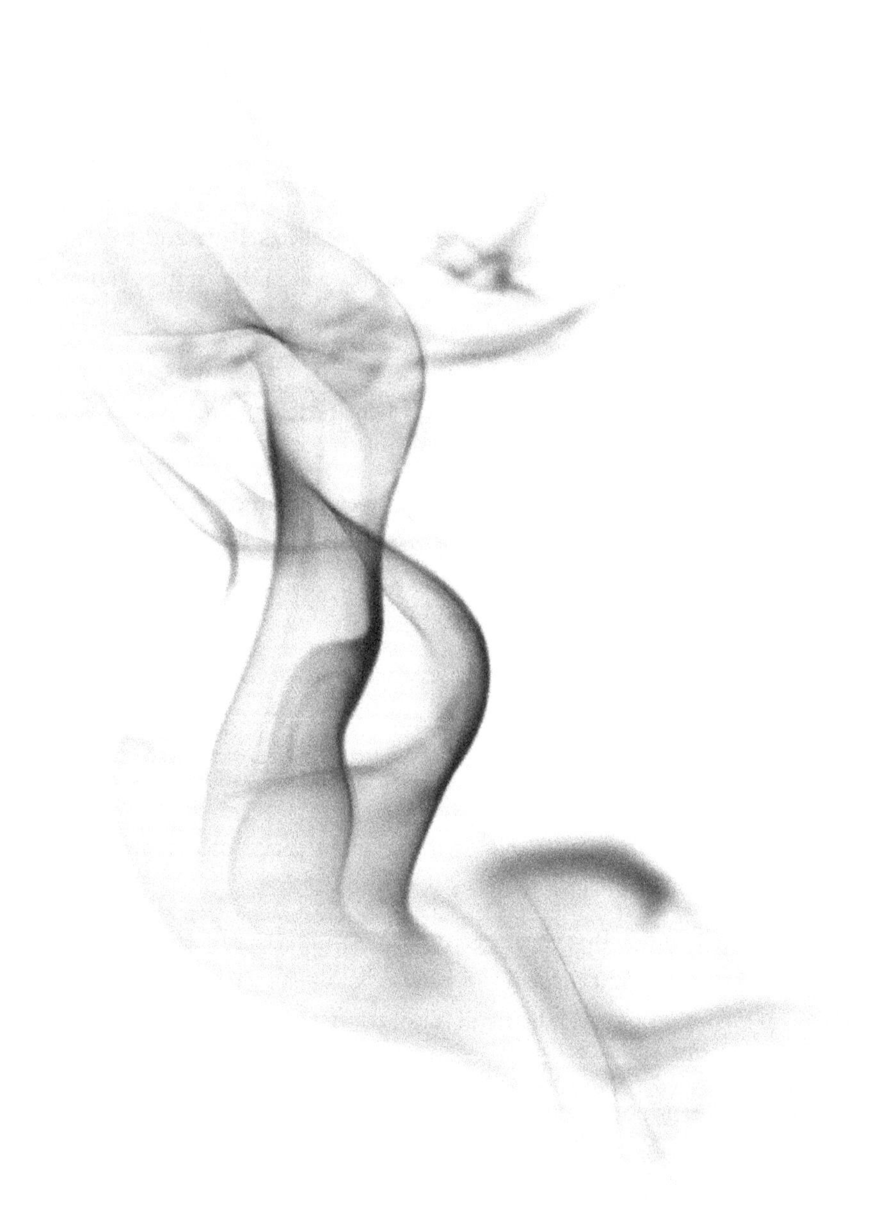

CHAPTER 5

Fantasies of Vape

As an interesting supplement to Dr. Tsai's and others' deep concerns regarding heat and inhalation, see below a **2011** review and description of one of the early generations of the Juul e-cigarette which they tout as NOT being an e-cigarette. They are especially clear to affirm that it has "clean vapor technology" because it does not produce tobacco or smoke but instead, uses BUTANE!! Ironically, this review appeared on the site www.electroniccigarettes.net.

The Ploom Vaporizer is the newest technology on the market available to consumers looking for a smoking alternative. For those smokers who are interested in "Switching, not Quitting," or if you are looking for a smoking alternative with most of the same benefits as well as a few others e-cigarettes have, but want something that isn't an electronic cigarette, the Ploom model One Vaporizer is just what you have been looking for.

The Ploom Vaporizer combines clean vapor technology and all natural tobacco "pods" to deliver nicotine into your system without ever actually burning the tobacco or producing smoke. Ploom is set apart from electronic cigarettes because Ploom does not require a battery for operation (it uses butane instead).

The model One's users can choose between 100% REAL U.S. grown & cured tobacco packed into tiny packages called "pods," or from an expanding line of "Herbal Pods," which are nicotine-free and contain a blend of herbs and natural flavorings that can actually freshen your breath like the intense Peppermint included in their "Kick-Ass Mint" Pod. We thought it would be a great idea to introduce Ploom to ECR's visitors to reach out to those that submitted user reviews claiming they have tried E-cigs but they just don't taste enough like an "analog" or traditional tobacco cigarette. For these people that want that authentic taste of real tobacco, we think Ploom will be an excellent alternative.

The Ploom model One Vaporizer is about the size of a pen, or a tipped cigarillo, and operates with a patented technology which uses butane to heat the tiny pods through Ploom's proprietary catalyst system. When the Ploom model One is filled with butane, it lasts for two hours of use before needing to be refilled. To quantify that, a regular tobacco cigarette takes four minutes to smoke (on average) and if you smoke 20 a day, that is an hour and a half. So the Ploom Vaporizer needs to be refilled with butane after the time you would have spent smoking 30 cigarettes. For those who smoke a pack a day outside, you can now switch to the Ploom Vaporizer alternative and have an extra hour and a half indoors :).

Each Ploom Pod lasts between 5-10 minutes, depending on the individual's habits after getting accustomed to using the Ploom. Another bonus is each Ploom Pod is 100% recyclable, so after it loses its flavor, you can recycle the Ploom Pod anywhere you recycle other metals, certainly this fact alone sets the Ploom far apart from tobacco cigarettes that produce a cigarette butt after each cigarette is smoked. We all know that cigarette butts are anything but recyclable and sight for sore eyes when littered throughout our cities and roadways.

Ploom offers two types of Pods with a current total of 7 varieties:

Tobacco Blends:

- Naked – taste of 100% pure tobacco

- Rocket – adds hot cinnamon and mint to natural tobacco

- Cafe Noir – a hint of cacao taste

- Gold – a hint of honey-cognac

- Orchard – natural tobacco combined with peach flavors

Herbal Blends:

- Kick-Ass Mint – natural peppermint flavor with breath-freshening appeal

- Blue Tea – English Breakfast Tea and berry flavors

Using the Ploom model One is simple, affordable and quite enjoyable! It is made right here in the U.S. in San Francisco, Calif., to a high quality standard. Ploom now offers a starter kit that comes with a choice of a 2-Pack Black Case or a 2-Pack White Case that will hold everything you need to take your Ploom from place to place and is small enough to fit into a pocket or purse. The only accessories you will most likely need are extra mouthpieces and butane, which are both offered below $5. With the cost savings and the flexibility of places that the Ploom Vaporizer can be used (anywhere e-cigarettes can be used), ECR.net highly recommends it to our readers.

This is a unique product that is the only of its kind, and after being an avid e-smoker for nearly 2.5 years now, I didn't think anything could lead me back to real tobacco! However, the cleanliness and robust flavors produced by the Ploom Vaporizer are a perfect treat for me when I want to take my taste buds to a place I've not yet been able to find with ANY other product, including the many e-cigarettes I've tried and ALL other forms of tobacco.

NOTE: This product is NOT an electronic cigarette. You are still able to use it everywhere you can use an e-cigarette, but it is based on hookah or shisha technology and is classified as a pipe tobacco product. Electronic cigarettes and the Ploom model One Vaporizer each have their own distinct and unique advantages and one is not better than the other. They are both great for their various applications and preference can only be obtained by trying each of them for yourself or reading the feedback by your peers below.

As reported by www.topclassactions.com, in 2015, the U.S. Food and Drug Administration (FDA) attempted to institute a ban on Juul pod flavors such as blueberry and mint, but were stymied by industry lobbyists. This is according to a *Los Angeles Times* review of thousands of pages of documents from the time, including the FDA's proposed new tobacco rules and records of lobbyists who met with administration officials prior to the decision to stop the ban from going into effect.

The ban, had it been allowed to go into effect, might have saved thousands, perhaps millions, of young people from developing nicotine addiction and prevented the hundreds of cases of lung disease that have been attributed to vaping in recent months. According to officials interviewed by the *LA Times,* the decision to strip the ban on Juul pod flavors from the FDA's proposal was based on a "cost-benefit analysis," indicating that the economic burden on retailers having to eliminate Juul pods and similar products was greater than the potential health risks.

In October 2015, a draft of the proposed rule warned of the "attractiveness of flavors, especially to youth and young adults, and the impact flavored tobacco products may have on youth initiation." This concern had already been noted by the Centers for Disease Control (CDC) a year earlier. Since 2011, the CDC had noted that e-cigarette use among middle and high school students had increased by 800 percent. When asked in a survey why they vaped, four-fifths of teens responded, "It comes in flavors I like."

As previously stated, the e-cigarette industry was taking a page from Big Tobacco's playbook. Despite this, Juul has published the following advertisement in order to distance itself from the tobacco companies:

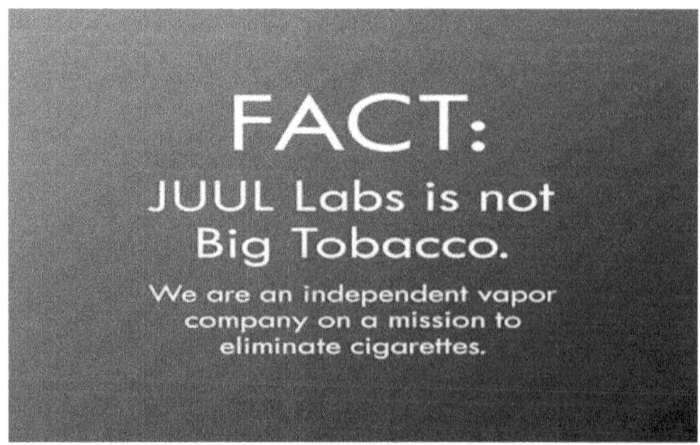

Consider additional information from the Reuters Investigation that confirms the progression, denial and negligence in an article by Chris Kirkham, paraphrased below. Keep in mind that any testing for safety is hard to find, but the safety considerations below, though minor anyway, were dismissed:

"FDA documents given to the White House warned that cigarette companies had used flavoring agents identical to those used in artificially-flavored candies – and when heated and concentrated, could be toxic. And yet, this scientific evidence was pushed aside. The FDA's proposed ban was widely supported by the scientific community as well as public health officials when it was submitted to the White House for approval in mid-October 2015. Two weeks later, the Office of Management and Budget (OMB) held the first in a series of over 100 meetings with business leaders, pro-industry representatives, and lobbyists, who over the next several months, drowned out public voices.

By the time all was said and done, when the final rule granting the FDA regulatory oversight was published in May 2016, the flavor ban had been stripped – along with all scientific documentation about the possible impact on youth. Instead, there was a vague statement in which the FDA said it was "seeking further data on the role of flavored products in youth initiation."

So, the question remains, did Juul pod flavors drive an epidemic? TobaccoFree Kids.org states the following:

"The youth e-cigarette epidemic is a public health emergency that demands the strongest possible action by the Food and Drug Administration and policy makers on all levels. The FDA has taken some steps to address this crisis, including announcing plans to restrict where certain flavored e-cigarettes are sold. But these plans don't go far enough. The Campaign for Tobacco-Free Kids and other public health groups have called on the FDA to do more, starting with a ban on the flavored products that have made e-cigarettes so popular with kids."

"Further, they concluded that 'the delay in reviewing the products before they hit the market deprives the public of critical information needed to make informed choices, contributes to confusion among smokers about the quality and safety of devices and permits the proliferation of products that are highly appealing to youth.'"

Consider this: In 1996, 36% of kids were smoking traditional cigarettes. Today, only 9% of these kids smoke. The war on cigarette smoking was won.

But, frighteningly, the use of vape pens by teens rose an unprecedented 78% between 2017 and 2018. And Juuls are delivering nicotine at higher levels and more effectively than any other e-cigarette. Remember, when initial versions of e-cigarettes were not delivering the spike of nicotine, Juul found a way to correct the "problem."

Mangoes and peaches and mint, oh my!

Now, two-thirds of teenagers believe that vape liquids contain only flavorings; only about 13 percent realize that it is a nicotine delivery system. Most teenagers are unaware of anything toxic in their e-cigarettes, yet new tests are uncovering a host of additional metals, or toxins, on top of the ones already mentioned by Dr. Tsai. These can be manganese or formaldehyde among others. And these toxins affect the neurological system. They can literally change your brain and how your body receives information from it. At www.drugabuse.gov, statistics indicate that 70 percent of teens are exposed to e-cigarette advertisements. It's important to highlight that e-cigarette use among youth exceeds the use of cigarettes and other tobacco products.

According to the National Youth Tobacco Survey (NYTS) released by the U.S. Centers for Disease Control and Prevention (CDC) and the Food and Drug Administration (FDA), e-cigarettes have been the most commonly-used tobacco product among youth since 2014. Five point three million youth were current e-cigarette users in 2019 — an increase of over 3 million students since 2017. Among high school students, e-cigarette use increased by 135 percent from 2017 to 2019, increasing from 11.7% to 27.5%. Among middle school students, e-cigarette use more than tripled from 2017 to 2019, increasing from 3.3% to 10.5%.

The same survey found that among those who had used e-cigarettes in the past 30 days, 34.2% of high schoolers and 18% of middle schoolers were frequent users of e-cigarettes, using e-cigarettes on at least 20 of the preceding 30 days. Twenty-one point four percent of high school e-cigarette users and 8.8% of middle school e-cigarette users were daily users, a strong indication of addiction. This amounts to 1.6 million middle and high school students who were frequent users of e-cigarettes, including nearly 1 million (970,000) daily users. Data from another national survey, the 2019 Monitoring the Future study, found that one out of nine high school seniors (11.7%) report that they vaped nicotine nearly daily.

Data from the 2016-2017 wave of the FDA's Population Assessment of Tobacco and Health (PATH) study found that 96.1 percent of 12- to 17-year-olds who had initiated e-cigarette use since the last survey wave started with a flavored product. Additionally, it found that 97 percent of current youth e-cigarette users had used a flavored e-cigarette in the past month and 70.3 percent say they use e-cigarettes "because they come in flavors I like." While the methodology is not comparable to the PATH study, the 2019 NYTS found that 57.3% of high school e-cigarette users use mint or menthol flavors, an increase from 38.1% in 2018. Among high school Juul users, mint is the most popular flavor.

Adult Use. Data from the National Health Interview Survey (NHIS) show that in 2018, 3.2 percent of adults currently used e-cigarettes every day or some days. (It was 2.8 percent in 2017, 3.2 percent in 2016 and 3.5 percent in 2015.)

Let's break down the numbers into shockingly simple terms. The ratio of youth users vs. adult users:

E-cigarette use is highest among younger adult populations. According to the 2018 NHIS, 7.6 percent of 18- to 24-year-olds currently use e-cigarettes every day or some days, an increase of 46.2% from 5.2% in 2017. Earlier data from the 2015 NHIS showed that 40 percent of young adult e-cigarette users had never been cigarette smokers, raising concerns that e-cigarettes may be attracting young non-smokers to tobacco use. Data from another survey, the 2016 Behavioral Risk Factor Surveillance System (BRFSS), estimates that 1.2 million young adult e-cigarette users are never cigarette smokers.

Social media has had a major role in addicting the youth of today. Again, on all the major social networking sites except www.HIVE80.com and in all the right "point of sale" locations, Juul implies that a cool, happy, connected lifestyle equals Juuling. So much so, that as so many teens have said, "Everyone's doing it." But, while those in charge of the CDC and FDA now characterize vaping use in the United States as "a teen epidemic," you have only to look at the UK to know why they have no vaping epidemic among teens. The reason? No advertising on social media is allowed. In addition, Britain puts a cap on the amount of nicotine allowed in e-cigarettes and guess what? It's half the amount allowed in the U.S. Not surprising to learn that they may actually have some success using vapes as Bowen and Monsees say they originally intended, to get cigarette smokers to quit smoking by using e-cigarettes; they are not trying to hook youth, but rather, help adults.

And for a while, the slick advertisements, the upscale events, the free samples and celebrity endorsements and cool packaging worked. The guerilla tactics worked, until they became the elephant in the room. The emergency room.

CHAPTER 6

When Our Child was Vaped, the Whole Family Suffered

As noted earlier, a teen in Michigan is the first to receive a double lung transplant. His story appears here. His is just one of the many sad vaping stories of heartbreak for patients and their families. At the risk of being tedious, I've included almost the entire GoFundMe page with updates to approximate the family's journey (which of course is impossible) as best as I can. I've also reversed the order to start at the beginning, so readers share the journey more in real time. As stated previously, sometimes we are removed from the personal reality of these tragic vaping events with phrases like "teen receives" or "vape explodes" or "schools warn." Life-altering consequences unfold in the day-to-day for patients and their families. Their fears, limitations, losses, financial hardships, and complications are personal and exhausting and unbearable. This family relies heavily on their faith for survival and hope. I hope as your read you can look past any differences and focus on what binds us all as mothers, fathers, sisters, brothers, extended family and in the family of humanity. And I ask that you join the McKnights and not turn away, no matter how unpleasant; sometimes that's the best we can do.

The story of Walker McKnight from his GoFundMe page

Walker is the son of Dave and Candy (Barnes) McKnight and is an incredible athlete on a cheerleading scholarship at Florida Atlantic University. In March of this year, he came down with what he thought was a common cold or maybe the flu. He decided to make the 2.5-hour drive home to Orlando so he could be home with his parents. Days after arriving home, his mom rushed him to the emergency room as he was having difficulty breathing. His mom, Candy, is a nurse so understands the gravity of breathing difficulty.

Walter was diagnosed with severe pneumonia Friday, March 8th, and put in the ICU. During his stay in the ICU, he was also diagnosed with multiple viruses including an adenovirus. He was extremely sick. His condition steadily deteriorated with his left lung collapsing from infection.

Doctors told the family on Friday, March 15th that he would likely not survive. His saving grace was his age and health. After 10 hours of trembling from fever on Saturday he asked to be intubated — he wanted to live but could not fight to breathe any more. On Sunday, the 17th, the infection spread to his right lung causing it to collapse as well. He was airlifted from Orlando Regional Medical Center to FL Hospital — as the family said their goodbyes to Walker, the hospital called the chaplain because they did not expect him to survive the short trip.

By the grace of God, he made the trip. He was rushed into surgery and put on ECMO, a form of life support, which oxygenated his blood and gave his lungs a much-needed rest. He ultimately spent 63 days on ECMO where survival rates are incredibly low — the average course of ECMO treatment is five days. In addition to the invasive ECMO treatment, he was on a feeding tube and lost use of his kidneys.

During his stay in the ICU, his doctors discovered that Walker, like many kids his age, had been "vaping," using Juul products. These deliver astoundingly high doses of nicotine (one e-liquid pod is equal to a pack of cigarettes), plus an array of chemicals. Doctors believe this contributed to his body's inability to recover. He was released from the ICU in late August and has had to return on three separate occasions due to breathing trauma. His left lung has never recovered and he is still on dialysis. He will ultimately have to endure a kidney and lung transplant.

His mother has to care for him full time, and his father is trying to manage paying bills and creating normalcy in their life for their daughter.

From the community:

"We have asked the community to help support them financially both for their day-to-day needs and long-term, mounting medical bills. Thank you in advance for your love, prayers, and financial help." #withyouwalker.

3/19 - Praise God Walker is doing better! He is still intubated and on ECMO but they were able to start flushing his lungs. His fever has come down from close to 105 to 101. Please keep praying.

3/20 - Nickie (Walker's aunt) spoke with the infectious disease doctor this morning. The doctor said that the adenovirus is the source of Walker's pneumonia.

Walker did have a good night, was able to rest, and his stats were stable. He still has fever and is fighting the infection, also still on ECMO and still intubated. Sherry (Walker's grandmother) has come down with this same virus and is in Orlando Regional Medical Center. The family is going back and forth to visit them both. Thanks to everyone for your support, love, and prayers. Obviously, they are much needed.

3/21 - Walker is stable and remains intubated on ECMO in ICU. His bone marrow was negative for cancer and his CT scan came back with no unexpected surprises. He is moving to every other day on his bronc washes and getting a tracheotomy tomorrow. He also continues to fight the adenovirus. Please keep praying, specifically for this virus to die off. Thanks to all.

3/22 - This morning they are performing a tracheostomy at his bedside that will allow them to remove the intubation tube and make him much more comfortable. We are very happy! Happy to have had two positive days in a row and confidently expecting a third day today. This will begin his march toward normalcy.

And march he will just as he used to do as a 3- to 4-year-old. Wearing his tall yellow rain boots, he would order his me maw, papa, and Nana to march! Making them follow him around the house in a line as he leads the way. :-) They just loved that.

3/23 - The team continues to lower the ventilator settings as well as sedation medication with the goal to try and slowly wake him up while finding balance between pain and anxiety. The chest X-ray is slightly better and he has not had a fever in three days. Today my heart is filled with hope. I sit by his bedside looking at his sweet face and I am filled with gratefulness to God and all his mercy and grace.

Wow "bronch" was great. Dr. Heim said it looks so much better in the lungs. He has no plans to "bronch" for the next two days

Again thank you all for being a part of this journey

The McKnight Family

3/24 - This is day 17 ICU and day 8 on ECMO...

The doc said his lungs are looking much better!! Slow and steady wins the race. All his vitals are good. They are keeping him sedated with a little bit of consciousness. Changing his meds to slowly bring him up to consciousness. No fevers which is great. And today when they moved him, he tolerated it much better than yesterday when his heart raced and pulse quickened. Today he handled it like the Champion that he is.

And the Champion he will become again through God's favor on his life.

Thanks be to God and his church (our family, friends, and supporters in Christ) that are supporting him through this very difficult time.

This will be the last update on GoFundMe site. For future updates please go to the post hope site. The link will be on Dave or Candy's Facebook page.

3/25 - This is day 18 in the ICU and day 9 still on ECM.

Today is a good day. I think the team has found the perfect combination of medications that will best support Walker as he continues to improve. His chest X-ray is looking better. The team even moved him into a chair today! This is another milestone. Yes, we are cautioned two steps forward and one step back but overall today is a win for us! Future updates will be on the post hope site below.

Link to post hope site: https://posthope.org/walkers-journey-home

3/28 - update by Auntie Gail

Well, the saying goes, one step forward and two steps back when dealing with ECMO. That should be translated to "days." We had a good day Monday, but today and yesterday have been difficult. As soon as we lower sedation to try to wake him, he gets anxious and fights his respirator and lines, raising his blood pressure and heart rate as he hyperventilates. Doctors say it could be 3-5 days of this. We thought he was making a turn Monday, but not yet. This is a difficult process to watch! Please pray for protection for his liver and kidneys. Pray that they can find the right combination of sedation, pain meds and anti-anxiety drugs to allow him to wake safely from his induced sleep. Pray for the McKnights to keep faith and hope in the days to come.

3-31 - Update by Dave (Dad)

The best news is that he is starting slowly to be more aware and responsive. We have made baby steps in the right direction, still very, very sick. His lung X-ray looked much better today than yesterday!! Please continue your prayers as they are keeping him afloat while his body heals. Our shared body of Christ is very strong and we are beyond thankful for all the support Walker and his family has received during this most difficult of days. The amazing thing is that this too shall pass and we will again be enjoying life together as family. Thanks be to God for what he is doing in our lives today, tomorrow, and always.

4-1-19 Update by Candy (Mom)

Day 25 ICU and day 15 ECMO. Every day I sit and watch my son battle for his life. Today things have been very slow and that is OK. He is tired and needs extra help today. I am reminded how delicate his life is as I look at all the machines and watch as this awesome team works diligently all day and night together to make sure Walker has everything he needs to live and get better. I am so grateful for their endless drive to provide excellent safe care to Walker.

4-5 - Update by Dave (Dad)

Dr. Swanson's (from First Presbyterian Church) anointing is working!! God is great!! Great seems so trivial when describing the God of the Universe that loves each of us like we love our own children, unconditionally.

Walker is on his way home. Day by day getting better and better. The ECMO team are true miracle workers in serving the very, very sick helping them to return to the living through expedient thoughtful care, using the best technology available. We are forever in their debt.

Just know today that Walker will be back with us in due time. He will once again be bringing his smile for life to many of you and more. Please pray for continued healing that no bacteria can enter his system. That he has a speedy recovery. Thank you!!

4/10 - Update by Dave (Dad)

We are on day 34 of ICU and day 24 on ECMO with many more ahead. But we are headed in the right direction — home :-).

In last few days, they have successfully reduced Walkers IV drips from eight major meds at beginning of his stay on the ECMO unit down to one IV drip today. Yesterday he stood up under his own weight for 1st time! :-) Baby steps. As we have heard, if he only got 1% better every day, he would be 100% better in 100 days.

On the Florida Hospital ECMO unit, slow and steady wins the race as they say here. And as we have learned, the lungs are called "lazy lungs" as they are the slowest to heal. His lungs are much better but still have a long road ahead. We (his family) have all been pitching in to help in so many ways, much thankful for our family and friends that have been supportive through all of these extraordinarily tough circumstances. Ever onward, ever forward we march!

4/19 - Update by Auntie Gail

33 days on ECMO.....

Today marks the end of a very tough week for Walker. Critical changes requiring six procedures including surgery. The days and weeks are flying by, as it has been six weeks since Walker began this journey in intensive care. He is hanging tough and taking things well. His regimen is to get moving and stand several times a day, resting in between. One of Walker's doctors said he hit "cruise control" today! Let's pray he cruises through the weekend with no extra difficulties. The medical staff in the ECMO unit continues to exceed all expectations in delivering his complex care! Have a blessed Easter weekend celebrating the Resurrection of our Savior and Lord!!

Our amazingly strong and beautiful daughter Laura dubbed Gail our MVP since these trials began. Never has there been a better Sister, Auntie, Sister-in-law, and friend than our Gail!! Her knowledge and support have been so critical throughout this ordeal. She truly is our MVP ♥

4/11 - Update by Dave and Candy

We had a consult today with a transplant pulmonologist, Dr. Kim, who informed us that it is a very real potential of a double lung transplant. It does not mean that it will happen but that it is a real possibility if his lungs do not improve. So please pray for a miracle that his lungs heal.

Our urgent goal right now is to get Walker moving within 10 days, standing on his own and starting to walk. This is important for two reasons, one that he recover strength and possibly get his lungs to heal, and two that he gather the strength to be eligible if he needs to have a transplant.

So pray for his lungs to heal and that he gets moving within next 10 days. On a good note, he is virus free so we do not need masks and gowns to visit him. He is more alert and aware. We are loving on him every day, praying over him, asking for healing graces. We have no choice but to hang tough through this incredible challenge. May God bless Walker with healed lungs and may God help him get up and get moving!! Love you all and thank you for your prayers

4/21 - Easter Sunday

We are very blessed to be under the cover of his wings, majestic wings that rose to a glory beyond all others to rule over heaven and earth, our Jesus! Today is our Super Bowl Sunday to celebrate the spirit of Christ being alive and among us. His spirit hovers over Walker keeping him Walker Strong as he faces the challenges ahead, challenges that he can overcome as he is lifted in prayer by many, many believers. Stay Walker Strong!!

His team of nurses have him right where He wants them, taking care of every need beautifully. He is blessed to have a strong team that is passionate about getting him up and moving with a steady daily therapy of standing, movements, and breathing postures. He stood for 10 minutes today and stayed off the ventilator for close to two hours!! We have had four good days in a row. Thank you, God.

Happy Easter to you all and please continue praying specifically for two things — supernatural healing of his right lung and that the spirit of Christ's peace of mind hover over his body. Together we are bringing Walker home. One day at a time through faith in our God that loves us as his own children. How sweet is that!!

4/22 - First Words!

"Hello," says Walker, his first word spoken yesterday since March 16th. Then he said, "I'm sorry" to nurse staff, I think for being difficult, so sweet. Today he said, "I love you all" to his mom, dad, grandma, and auntie all watching him in rapt attention during his second day of speech therapy.

Physically, he is progressing daily by standing, movements, and breathing therapy. Getting a little better each day. One of the hardest things to get set right is his medication as there are many different goals to manage at once. We had some challenges with this over the weekend but have made changes since then that have improved his condition.

Dr. Swanson was kind to stop in today to pray over Walker and to hug his mom that needs lots of love ♥ right now. His family got together last night to share in a meal, some laughs, and fellowship of prayer. To say this situation has affected his entire family greatly would be an understatement and unfairly exclude the effect this has had on his greater community of friends and family that are praying for him daily.

His mom and dad would like to personally thank the member of the Christian group "12 Ordinary Women" that stopped by today and blessed Candy generously. Thank you! The journey home continues....

April 30th - Day 44 on ECMO: Here is situation:

The family has been told that patients who stay on ECMO more than 40 days have a greatly reduced survival rate. The doctors are going to begin a transplant evaluation next week in preparation for potential surgery as a safety net for his condition. Currently, he is not a candidate for transplant until they can get him walking and in better health. The video is from Saturday. You can see the pain and desperation in Walker's face, knowing that living through extreme pain right now is his only way to heal.

Dave said he saw Walker for the first time uncovered from the waist up and it "took his breath away." He knew there were all sorts of tubes and other life saving measures but found it both crushing and amazing all at once the extent of medical intervention to save a person's life.

Candy lost her job at the end of Nov '18 due to reorganization and had not yet found another one when all of this began. Dave has an insurance business where he is compensated on commissions of sales only. Their only income is coming from the few sales that Dave's been able to muster during this catastrophic time. Many of you have emailed and asked how you can continue to help. Walker needs his parents by his side, pushing him to walk, to talk, and to fight for his life.

I cannot imagine trying to work when my son needed me more than he ever had or ever will. They are looking at three or more months of hospital time and recovery time to come home (God willing). Then rehab from home for months following.

The Need: Their basic monthly needs are approximately $5,000 per month. I would love for this powerful community of supporters to raise an additional $15,000 to get them through the next three months so their sole focus can be on Walker's healing and survival. If you are able to donate a second time that is wonderful; if not please share this story with as many people as possible. Thank you.

From Dave: We are very thankful for all of our friends, and people we have never met, who have generously given their love, time, prayers, and money. Walker's aunts have graciously taken on the responsibility for Laura's school cost.

It does indeed take a village and we could not do this without all of you!

May 1st - Day 45 on ECMO

A day in the life of Walker: he was only able to sleep three to four hours at a time, as the medical team wakes him by checking his blood gas percentage as it effects the sweep of his ECMO machine (meaning they measure the percentage of oxygen and carbon dioxide) which oxygenates his blood while pulling off the carbon dioxide build up. Then it takes at least three nurses to prepare him to stand, which he has been doing three, sometimes four, times a day in an effort to get him moving as moving is key to getting off this machine. They are shifting him from side to side constantly throughout the day to lessen potential of beds sores. He has one tough one on his tailbone that they are working at getting better cause this hurts his sitting position. His mom has been really helping to push ahead his rehab by continuing the moves throughout the day that his physical therapy team puts him through once a day.

His respiratory therapy has been pushing him hard to breathe through his trachea on his own (called spontaneous) as much as he can, usually five to six hours at a time when they first started. The purpose is to get his lungs working and breathing on his own. This is essentially what a workout would be for you and me. His constant refrain being "I can't breathe" is normal because they say it feels to him like he is on the edge of drowning even though his oxygenation performance is good overall.

The goal right now is to improve his lung performance so that he can be removed from the ECMO machine. It's a complicated process that involves lots of science having to do with him sustaining himself without support and they won't take him off it till they have observed him for days successfully breathing/oxygenating on his own.

Thank you for your support so that his family can stay by his side.

May 2nd - Day 46 on ECMO

Walker took a step back today...he is now back on the vent with O2 increased from 28% to 60% and the ECMO sweep has gone from 1 up to 9. His lungs got tired and began to retain CO2 throughout the night. As the refrain goes on the ECMO unit, "two steps forward one step back is still a step forward." It's an easy cliche to say but much harder to actually live it, especially at this level of intensity.

While the work that is done on this unit, ECMO CVICU at Advent Health is cutting edge and one of best in the country and has saved Walker's life, but it is still a very hard process to watch for the parents/family members and very hard on the patients as well. We would say brutal, in fact. But worth every tough minute when you consider the alternatives. Five years ago this type of treatment did not exist and this ECMO unit is only 18 months old.

What it is like to be Walker's parents (from Dave):

Being Walker's parents right now is a complicated balancing act between taking care of him and trying to take care of yourself, between staying positive and strong for Walker and managing a deeply painful aching heart, between managing the sometimes overwhelming level of care he needs, and managing the business of your life. One thing I do know is that this has changed all of us in ways we will only discover down the road. Today we ask for prayer specifically that Walker's lungs will continue to improve and that his kidneys will restart when the timing is right. Protect him Lord from all bacteria, virus, and disease so that they will die upon touching his body. Thank you Father for today, tomorrow, and what you will do in the future for Walker.

Please continue to share this site as we are still a bit short of our goal. A step backwards means more hospital time. Thanks to all of you for loving this family!

May 3rd - Day 47 on ECMO

It's still a monumental battle to get Walker off of the ECMO machine under his own lung support. The tricky thing is the oxygen and carbon dioxide balance. Wednesday night while operating with minimal support his lungs underperformed regarding the throw off of carbon dioxide out of the system. So they had to up his support yesterday to compensate accordingly. The staff had been pushing Walker hard as he was improving each day for seven days in a row.

Today his stats are improving again heading back to levels they were before Wednesday, with some minor complications. Of course the complications don't feel minor to Dave & Candy when all they desperately want is to move their precious child out of ICU. He has a low-grade fever in response to the same bacteria that affected him a few weeks back, which was presumed to have been eliminated with standard antibiotics. So not the worst of situations, but it slows down his progress in the meantime.

From Dave:

Still in the forest not in the woods looking for a path out to greener fields. We will overcome through the grace of God alone. We are all helpless in situations like this clinging to a single vine for hope. Christ is our vine and he is stronger than we can fathom. Our human frailty is so evident at times like this where our efforts are reduced to hope. No matter how hard we try, we cannot fix this. And that is what we are left with at the end of our crying out in prayer.

Please pray that God continues to heal Walker and to strengthen his body and mind for the road ahead of him and us. His journey is turning out to be epic by normal standards. And we will have an epic comeback by Walker in his time. Our hope lies with Christ alone.

Thanks to all who continue to support. We are nearing our fundraising goal so please continue to share this site. As you can see, this will be a very long road to recovery.

May 4th - Day 48 on ECMO

Walker is fighting an infection, has a fever, stats are dropping, ECMO is up, starting dialysis now instead of tonight. Please pray for God to kill this infection now, and for protection and healing of his lungs. He did stand and shuffled a few steps, which is good, but we need this infection to go away now!

From Dave:

A snapshot of a day in our current life: yesterday

I awake at 6 a.m., dogs barking as back door opens, Candy coming home early from an unsuccessful attempt at staying the night with Walker. Sleeping overnight in the hospital has been my job and I sleep there pretty well overall, considering. I'm up to walk the dogs while Candy gets a couple of hours sleep then I'm off to the hospital to meet Auntie Gail and a minister for prayer and counsel.

While in the meeting, I text a quick note to Candy asking her to take some time to pray, to gather some strength, and refresh. She immediately calls asking what is going on as she thought (lack of sleep) I meant pray now for Walker and she panicked. I had to talk her off the cliff, but to no avail as she heard his updated stats and was very upset! I decided heading home now was best to be beside her as we have to stick together when one of us is krumping (as they say in our world).

On my way out I spot Alex, an awesome chaplain at Florida Hospital, and ask him to pray with me as prayer seems to be the only thing that helps get through the day. At home Candy is pissed and very mad at God, which I can totally understand. As she says, when will these days in the valley end! How can he be doing this to Walker? His care has gone beyond brutal into cruelty from what we see. We hold each other trembling in angst. What next?

Candy showers and gets dressed to head back to the hospital with me early afternoon. I know her being with Walker is the only cure at this moment. We did not speak a word on the way there. Seeing Walker is good because his face is bright and his eyes so blue and he is talking. His voice has gotten much stronger in a few days talking with the trach device. After a few minutes a nurse pops in to tell us we have a visitor, Pastor Becky Davis from First Presbyterian Church.

We sit with Becky, who of course is a God send at that moment for Candy, and they talk about the reality of being mad at God. She commiserates in understanding saying it's I-4 these days that tends to push her buttons. She says "God appreciates our pain and can handle whatever we throw at him," even literally. We head into Walker's room and Becky prays with us over him.

We spend a couple of hours with Walker as he has a fever so bundled up tight and resting. Then we tell him we are going out for a bite and will be back after. He asks that we not be long and to hurry back. I decide a familiar place is best and we go to one of our favorites, Firebirds, right around corner. At 7 p.m. on Friday night, as luck would have it, we walked right in and our favorite table was open. Sweet! Ahh, the little things. We agree that food doesn't really taste like much right now and that we really can't focus on any other subject than Walker.

We decide at dinner that my suggestion to move my office into back of house where Walker's room is now and to move him up to front bedroom with larger windows and easier access for us is best. This lightens our mood a bit with the hope of him coming home. Our dinner is very good, cocktails even better, then we head back to hospital. Sticking together helps us both feel a little bit better.

We get to Walker's room and he is awake and we meet his night nurse. At night they tend to rotate his nursing more than the days where he gets a fairly familiar rotation. He asked us for first time, "Why me?" Which is great because we see him improving his thought process beyond simple commands of pain, cold, nausea and the like. No easy answer of course. He also starts talking about the food channel saying he likes the Greek grape leaf thing with hummus :-). Again, we love to hear him talk about this as it shows he is getting better, getting hungry for some real food!

We tell him it is time that we cannot stay at night anymore as the docs and family have recommended we give him space and get better rest for days ahead. He asks me to stay, but I say no and he wants us to promise to come early. This he repeats several times before we leave. We head out doing the blue mile shuffle back to our car in silence. Our roller coaster day is coming to an end off to bed to do it again today. And the beat goes on....

Day 59 in ICU and day 49 on ECMO

News Flash!! Just got a call from Candy that Walker just walked about 44 ft for his 1st time out!! Woop Woop Woop! Now we really have a reason to celebrate Cinco de Mayo! Walker's fever is gone and he has stood several times already. They had to do a couple of little procedures to include re-stitching his ECMO line and pulling his chest tube out 3 cm. Most people are eating tacos and drinking margaritas and we are celebrating a few steps across a room — and so grateful to be able to do so.

September 1, 2019

Walker had made it home as you all know. He sadly had to return to the ICU on Thursday the 28th. It has been a very traumatic and exhausting week for the McKnights. Walker had an infection that had been building up in his right lung and one doctor said it may be that his lung is giving out but they are not sure. The current diagnosis is not certain but what is certain is that his breathing has not gotten better but worse, it seems. Even if Walker recovers, again, he will be in rehab for at least 6 months, requiring 24-hour-a-day care by Dave and Candy. Dave is back to work as much as he can, but there is a delayed income factor in the annuity business. They are asking for your continued prayers and for financial donations. They have exhausted previous funds to get Walker home and we will now need further support to aid in his recovery until Dave's income is steady once again. We greatly appreciate your love and support.

Thanks again for all of you who have helped support this journey! All future updates will go through https://posthope.org/walkers-journey-home/journal/248835/5-6.

The family is of course wanting his stats to return as quickly as possible to where they were Monday/Tuesday last week when the ECMO team was talking about the possibility of getting him off ECMO. This fever set him back a few days but we are back on track gaining ground each day to get out of ICU period.

Together we lift up this prayer expectantly knowing God is at work healing Walker for his journey home!! Thank you all for your continued love and support!!

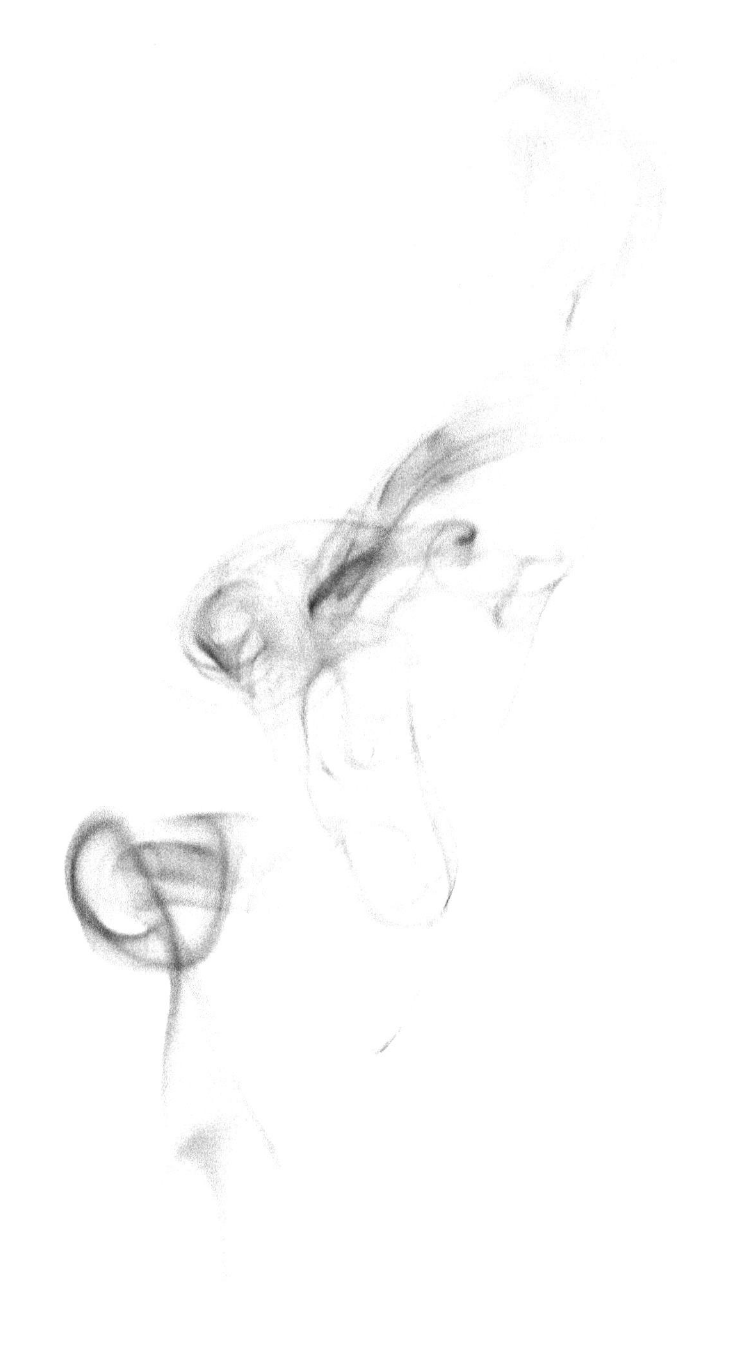

CHAPTER 7

Gang Vape

Circumstance and opportunity provide the basis for so many unplanned and uncontrollable events. While it may be that the founders of Juul started out innocently enough, simply looking for a novel and exciting project for a graduate thesis, as so often happens, money, excitement and ego can propel a project too quickly or without enough thought and research, and can take innocence into something darker, something less responsible and sadly, even dangerous. Even if the initial intent was not to harm, it seems as if the production of Juul took on a life of its own. Years ago there was the case of the Central Park jogger, and the crime was said to have been committed by the Central Park 6, who have since been exonerated. At the time, a theory of "wilding" was prominent in the discussion of how six fairly ordinary teens could turn into monsters. The science of group dynamics were forefront, focusing on how a group will sometimes commit atrocities that each of the individuals never would. Is that what happened here? Did Bowen and Monsees start out as "good kids" but become swept up in Big Tobacco themselves? Dazzled by a momentum of money and investors? Could be. Even if that's the explanation, it's doubtful that it matters to the victims or their families. Whatever the reason, the deed was done.

The following is taken from in the United States District Court, District of New Jersey:

Three NJ teens are suing Juul and their investors, (Defendants) contending the firm's e-cigarettes are a danger to vapers. In a proposed class-action suit, a Voorhees boy (Plaintiff) argues that he became addicted to nicotine when he started vaping at age 14. The suit seeks damages for all New Jersey residents "who have purchased, used, become addicted to or been otherwise harmed" by Juul's e-cigarettes.

Another plaintiff is a bright 19-year-old who has developed severe nicotine addiction and related health effects both known and unknown as a result of Defendants' orchestrated efforts to addict a new generation of teenagers to nicotine. Plaintiff continues to be severely addicted to nicotine, and this addiction will burden the remainder of her life. Defendants' wrongful conduct in marketing, promoting, manufacturing, designing, distributing, and selling Juul substantially contributed to Plaintiff's life-altering and permanent injuries. Two product-liabilities suits were brought by two other college students who say they began vaping as minors.

The suit contends that in 2015, Juul set out to recapture the magic of the most successful product ever made — the cigarette. Due to regulations and court orders preventing the major cigarette manufacturers from marketing to young people, youth smoking had decreased to its lowest levels in decades. While the public health community celebrated this decline as a victory, Juul saw an opportunity. Seizing on regulatory inaction and loopholes for e-cigarettes, Juul set out to develop and market a highly addictive product that could be packaged and sold to young people. Youth is and has always been the most sought-after market for cigarette companies, because they are the most vulnerable to nicotine addiction and are most likely to become customers for life. Juul was designed perfectly for teenagers. It does not look or smell like a cigarette. It is a sleek, high-tech, youth-friendly, battery-powered device in fun flavors like mango and cool mint, delivering powerfully potent doses of nicotine, along with aerosol and other toxic chemicals into the lungs, body and brain. Unlike noxious cigarette smoke, when a Juul user exhales, the smoke is undetectable. Juul is small, easily concealable and can be used practically anywhere without parents or teachers knowing; just Google "Juul in school" and find more than 23,000 videos on how to Juul anywhere without detection. This is part of the appeal, fostered and bolstered by Juul's viral marketing campaigns using young models to make the products look cool and stylish.

Defendants designed Juul to quickly and severely addict young people to nicotine, one of the most addictive chemicals in the world. By studying cigarette industry archives, Juul learned how to manipulate the nicotine in its products to maximize addictiveness, particularly among new users and young people, and thereby increase sales. Juul designed its products to have maximum inhalability, without any "throat hit" or irritation that would serve as a natural deterrent to new users. The sole purpose of this design element was to initiate new smokers, since those who already smoke cigarettes are tolerant to the throat hit sensation and associate it with smoking and nicotine satisfaction.

At the same time, Juul designed its device to deliver substantially higher concentrations of nicotine per puff than traditional cigarettes and most other e-cigarettes. This combination of ease of inhalation and high nicotine delivery makes Juul both powerfully addictive and dangerous.

Nicotine is particularly dangerous to young people, like Plaintiff, whose brains are still developing through the mid-20s. Nicotine is not only addictive to developing adolescent brains, but it also induces seizures and it permanently alters the structure of the brain and causes permanent mood changes and other cognitive disorders. Several studies, including one recently released by the American Stroke Association, have shown that e-cigarettes increase the risk of stroke, heart attack and coronary artery disease.

Other studies have shown that e-cigarettes containing nicotine significantly increase blood pressure, heart rate and arterial stiffness, and also cause vascular damage, which can lead to strokes and other cardiovascular injuries. These studies build on the well-established research that nicotine increases blood pressure. The United States Surgeon General has concluded that e-cigarettes, including Juul, are not safe for anyone under age 26. Even though e-cigarettes are unsafe for anyone under 26, Juul heavily promoted its products to young people. Following the wildly successful playbook laid out in historic cigarette industry documents, Defendants leveraged social media and utilized other marketing and promotion tactics, long outlawed for cigarette companies, to capture the highly-lucrative youth market. Juul preyed on youth using mediums and themes that exploit teenagers' vulnerabilities to e-cigarettes, even as reports linked them to higher risk of stroke, heart attack, diseased arteries (Jan. 30, 2019) creating and sustaining nicotine addiction, all for financial gain, and without giving kids any warnings about the serious risks of addiction, stroke, and other permanent injuries.

At the time Plaintiff used Juul none of Juul's advertising, marketing, promotion, packaging or website disclosed any of the health effects and risks that Juul knew or should have known would occur from use of its products. These risks include severe nicotine addiction, significant increases in blood pressure, vascular damage, increased risk of stroke, heart attacks and other cardiovascular injuries, permanent brain changes, mood disorders, heightened risk of cancer, seizures and other harms. Juul never disclosed that its products were unsafe for anyone under age 26. Instead, the imaging, advertising, promotion, packaging and overall marketing represented the product as safe, fun, and not harmful As one of the Juul founders has said:

"We don't think a lot about addiction here because we're not trying to design a cessation product at all...anything about health is not on our mind."

Juul's design, manufacturing, marketing and distribution of this product has proven this statement to be true. Since 2015 when Juul hit the market, Juul has become pervasive in schools across the country and adolescent use is rampant. Juul not only dominates the multi-billion-dollar e-cigarette market, it has expanded the size of that market significantly — mostly via young non-smokers. Defendant Altria (formerly known as Philip Morris) acquired a 35% stake in Juul for $12.8 billion, giving Defendant Altria access to the new generation of customers Juul has groomed.

Juul has created an epidemic, according to Alex Azar, the Secretary of the U.S. Department of Health and Human Services, "We have never seen use of any substance by America's young people rise as rapidly as e-cigarette use is rising." Juul's conduct has led to a surge in teen e-cigarette use, creating the "largest ever recorded [increase in substance abuse] in the past 43 years for any adolescent substance use outcome in the U.S." In a mere two years, Defendant undid more than a decade of progress in reducing teen smoking, thereby increasing nicotine use among teenagers to levels not seen since the early 2000s. Plaintiff was both a target and a victim of Juul's conduct. As a result of Defendants' conduct, Plaintiff has suffered life-altering personal injuries and seeks all appropriate remedies and relief.

And in *Forbes:*

A Connecticut man is suing Juul Labs for causing him to suffer a massive stroke after he became addicted to the company's products as a teenager. The case marks the first time the e-cigarette company has been sued for a medical issue this severe.

Maxwell Berger, 22, developed an addiction to Juul products during the summer of 2015 as he was finishing his last year of high school, the lawsuit says. By 2017, Berger was taking puffs of his Juul as often as every ten minutes, causing him to go through two cartridges every day. That July, Berger had a massive hemorrhagic stroke, which required three brain surgeries and more than 100 days in the hospital, the lawsuit states. It left him with "catastrophic and permanent injuries" such as left side paralysis, speech impairment and a 50% loss of vision from both eyes.

Law firms that we work with have won class action suits against large corporations and big verdicts against tobacco companies. These firms accused Juul of wrongful conduct that led to Berger's injuries. Specific charges include fraudulent concealment and intentional misrepresentation of the products and their risks, as well as negligence in promoting and selling to young people under age 26.

The suits paints Berger and others as one of the many teenagers who succumbed to Juul's viral marketing that made it seem "fun, healthy and cool." When Berger first tried it, the device had already "become ubiquitous among his high school friends," the suit claims. Within weeks, he had developed nicotine addiction and would take restroom breaks during family dinners in order to take a hit from his Juul, a battery-powered device which looks like a USB drive and converts a nicotine-based liquid into vapor for inhalation. The company previously said that each cartridge, or "pod," contains the same amount of nicotine as a pack of cigarettes, but it has since removed that information from its website.

Juul is intended as an alternative to cigarettes for adult smokers only, spokesman Ted Kwong told *Forbes* in a statement. "We do not want non-nicotine users, especially youth, to ever try our product. To this end, we have launched an aggressive action plan to combat underage use as it is antithetical to our mission. To the extent these cases allege otherwise, they are without merit and we will defend our mission throughout this process."

Stories on Instagram are plentiful.

In Florida, 19-year-old Chance Ammirata, who started vaping at 16, writes about his experience with a collapsed lung. He describes his experience as absolutely insane and life-changing. He's completely "negative mad" at the world and scared of how things will turn out. But he's turning his negativity into a drive to help others and get the message across so no one else has to go through what he did. In his own words,

"Change your mindset and throw out your Juul. I hope you realize that enough is enough and that nicotine is rotting our brains and destroying our bodies. It overcame me with emotions. I've never been happier to make such a difference. My surgery to get my chest tube removed is scheduled in around 2-3 hours and I'm insanely nervous. But I want to make sure my story is always out there and that the change doesn't stop. Every day we need to fight to help not only ourselves, but the ones we love to put down the nicotine. This epidemic has taken enough. We don't need more evidence telling is just how bad it is. How many more kids have to get hospitalized for us to stop!? None should be the answer. Don't take this with a grain of salt. And keep on pushing yourselves to take control of these cravings. I know it's hard and I know it will be a long 1-2 weeks of getting over the addiction. But 1-2 weeks is so much more worth it than a lifetime of consequences. #lunglove #stopJuul #revolution #wewillmakeachange #wearenotcontrolled"

And in Connecticut, Cara Fraser told BuzzFeed News that she was nervous to post on Instagram about the time she was placed in a medically-induced coma for seven days because, at age 19, she couldn't breathe on her own. She tells BuzzFeed she had originally only told family and close friends that it was likely her Juuling habit that put her there, but after seeing reports about other people being hospitalized with vaping-related lung injuries she felt like she should do something. "I just really wanted to help one person," said Fraser, who started vaping when she was 17. "Not only was it hard physically, it was very hard mentally to go through that. I didn't want anyone else to go through it."

Instead, she helped a lot more than just one person. Since posting her story on Facebook and Instagram on Sunday, at least nine people have reached out to her saying that she helped them quit. "When people tell me that I'm like — even if I don't know them — I'm just proud of them," the 21-year-old Fairfield, Connecticut, resident said. "It's definitely not the easiest thing to do...it kind of left me speechless."

In a story out of California, Fabian Castillo had decided to use vaping to deal with anxiety. And for a while it worked. He describes the nicotine as "masking" his stress. He had no idea e-cigarettes could be dangerous. Then, suddenly, he started to have breathing issues. Within days he was at the hospital being intubated and placed on a ventilator. "I looked at myself and I saw the stress that I was putting my mother through and I just don't want to see anybody go through that. I want people to look at me and use me as an example and picture them in that situation."

Castillo said the experience of nearly dying has caused him even more anxiety and forced him to take a break from school, work, and singing. Like Cara, he, too, was in a medically-induced coma for nine days which he said felt like nine months. He is now taking a semester off.

"I just feel so behind; everything was just put to a pause because I made that decision because I just started vaping. I didn't want anyone else to go through it and put their life on pause because they wanted to vape."

In the BuzzFeed News article, both Ammirata and Fraser said that they had only vaped Juul pods, which they bought at gas stations and smoke shops. Castillo said he had a SMOK e-cigarette and primarily used nicotine cartridges from smoke shops; however, he occasionally vaped THC cartridges provided by a relative.

Cara Fraser said that even after she was put in a coma for respiratory failure last year, she had a hard time quitting vaping. In December 2018, she started Juuling again and the breathing difficulties came roaring back. Now she's done for good.

"After the first time, I should have been like, what am I doing? But it's so addicting. It's just very hard to stop."

Tragedies abound from coast to coast:

In the San Francisco Bay area, a 45-year-old woman died of her pulmonary issues in November, six months after taking up vaping. Previously in good health, Amanda Arconti went from what she thought was just a bad cold and cough to acute respiratory distress. The *San Francisco Chronicle* reports that doctors often interview a patient about vaping these days, but that Arconti died so quickly, they didn't have the chance. She was almost immediately on a breathing machine in the ICU. Although the medical examiner won't rule conclusively that vaping was the cause of death, public health officials have tracked the symptoms, illnesses and deaths and have no reservations about the diagnosis. Pointing to "large numbers of patients with severe respiratory disease and lung injuries," they state that "the only common denominator was vaping."

In New York, 22-year-old Gregory Rodriquez checked into a hospital ER with a fever, vomiting and diarrhea. He felt unable to breathe but had no idea vaping could be the cause of how sick he felt. As reported in several news outlets, Gregory was "on the brink of death" and in less than 48 hours was hooked up to an artificial lung and being considered for a double lung transplant. Reportedly his lungs had filled with a thick, custard-like substance that was lodged in his restricted and inflamed airways. Oxygen was not getting to his bloodstream. The doctors at Northwell Health who treated them said he was "within hours of dying," He, too, ended up on the ECMO machine as a last resort. It saved him. Although he was in a medically-induced coma for three days, he returned home after only 12 days, which doctors reported as amazing compared to five other similar and serious cases they'd treated.

Going forward, Gregory is still working "not to think about vaping." He doesn't feel he is physically addicted, but is still dealing with the pull of the habit and cravings, especially for marijuana. His habit was costly in so many ways. As he says about buying cartridges for e-cigarettes, legally and "on the dark web," "Basically, it's Amazon, but for drugs."

And while he feels much better and is no longer breathless all the time, his doctor reports that his lung capacity is reduced by 60%.

CHAPTER 8

This year's hot accessory? A VTD!
(Vaping Transmitted Disease).

ALL the Juul kids have one!

So far we've seen just a few examples of teens suffering from VTDs. In Walter's story, Carly's story, Chance's, Fabian's, Cara's, Max's, and the lawsuits of three teens from New Jersey, the physical fallout from vaping is epidemic and as of yet to even be quantified in terms of what's to come for these individuals in later years.

"Not only does vaping pose serious health issues, such as damage to your heart and lungs, it can cause other physical changes that are very undesirable," says Ali S. Raja, MD, executive vice chairman of the department of emergency medicine at Massachusetts General Hospital and an associate professor at Harvard Medical School. He writes in *Parade* magazine about the potential for hair loss, skin changes, yellow teeth, no teeth, nervous affect, and smell.

In addition, a more severe of the lesser side effects is called "Vape Tongue."

Here are some other stories describing some of these lesser known but emerging medical issues and the unknown potential of their impact:

Vape Tongue

In an article for www.insider.com, Julia Naftulin reports that vaping teens are dealing with a side effect called "vape tongue," and doctors still don't know the long-term consequences. Citing a study in The Wall Street Journal, the article talks about the way the juices or solvents in the vaping liquid coat the tongue and desensitize it so the taste buds in the tongue can't receive flavor signals. Kind of ironic considering the lengths that some vape companies have gone to in order to add flavor to their products. Although "vape tongue typically resolves on its own when the vaper stops using for a few weeks," it's not known whether or not this side effect has long term consequences as it hasn't been studied.

It's important to note "vape tongue" shows up no matter what the vaper is using, be it nicotine or THC, because the condition is directly related to the solvents. Some of these solvents are propylene glycol, ethylene glycol, and vegetable glycerin. YUM, sounds delicious, right?

The theory is that the solvents, so necessary to deliver the vaped substance in an aerosol form, have this numbing effect with consistent use. They are also inflammatory to the nasal canal and interfere with the sense of smell, so necessary to the sensation of taste.

It's been reported that the deadening of taste not only affects the flavors of the vape, but also the individual's ability to taste food and beverages.

What about the effect on oral health? Gums? Teeth? No one knows for sure. No research currently exists but it's possible that, similar to smoking tobacco, there may be long-term problems in this area as well.

"In a study done as early as November of 2016, researchers found that after just a few minutes of puffing on both tobacco- and menthol-flavored vapes, oral tissue became inflamed, which can make someone more susceptible to oral diseases like gum disease or oral cancer. A follow-up study published in February found that vaping can change oral tissue on a molecular level, which could in turn increase cancer risk."

For these reasons, Dr. Erich Voigt, a clinical associate professor in the Department of Otolaryngology at NYU Langone Health, recommends vape users gradually wean off their devices and eventually swear off vapes entirely.

"My gut instinct is there will be long-term health consequences with continued use of vaping," Voigt said.

Hair Loss

Dr. Raja says that "because vaping can cause the same kinds of damage that smoking regular cigarettes can, when you vape, the smoke can damage your hair follicles, causing the possibility of hair loss. Research shows that this kind of hair loss can be super hard to treat, too, so your hair loss could be permanent."

In 2018 a study at the University of North Carolina Medical Center found that underestimating the negative effects of vaping is a bad idea. The study was led by Ilona Jaspers, professor of pediatrics, associate professor of microbiology and immunology, and director of the UNC Toxicology Program with a joint appointment at the UNC Gillings School of Global Public Health.

Jaspers has been a featured expert in several national media outlets, including *The New York Times,* for her research on the health effects of e-cigarettes.

She describes her job as safeguarding the public with regards to new products, and is always skeptical about unregulated products. She states that they know for certain that e-cigarettes change the inside of the lungs but that there are no studies to estimate what the long-term damage will be. A main problem is the change in proteins that occurs that may cause diseases that take years to develop. She talks about the flavors, which as substances are not the major problem. But she does note that while most or all of the flavors found in e-cigarettes may be approved by the FDA, we must remember that these have been approved for *ingestion*, not *inhalation.*

Of most concern with adolescents, she states, is Juuling. When they talk to her about starting Juuling, it is from scratch, as a new habit. These teens and young adults are not switching from cigarette smoking; they are picking up vaping as a new habit. Jaspers is adamant that the comparison people are making is false in terms of if e-cigarettes are safer than cigarettes because the comparison should be, are e-cigarettes safer than NO smoking of any kind? Because that's what's truly happening with teens.

What the UNC team found in a study about how vaping affects the e-smoker on a cellular level was striking. Cigarette smoking decreases the gene expression of **53** virus-fighting and bacteria-fighting genes. Vaping affects **358** of them. In terms of hair loss, "smoking has always been linked, but inconclusively. However, as a known unhealthy pursuit, it could contribute to biological deficiencies that manifest as thinning hair. The new evidence suggests that something similar could be true when people choose electronic cigarettes over traditional ones."

An interesting addition to the hair loss discussion is taking place in London at The Belgravia Centre hair loss clinics and at similar treatment centers in the U.S. Consider the following from the Limmer Center in San Antonio, Texas.

"At its core, e-cigarettes are nicotine delivery systems. Nicotine is a very addictive stimulant that has been found to damage your body in a number of ways.

e-cigarettes heat a solution of nicotine, flavoring, additives, and other chemicals for you to consume. Since the FDA doesn't currently regulate e-cigarettes, there are various amounts of nicotine found in electronic cigarettes depending on the brand you buy from, along with other potentially unrecorded chemicals." A study presented at the Society for Research on Nicotine and Tobacco 18th Annual Meeting found that e-cigarettes delivered similar levels of nicotine as tobacco cigarettes.

Unfortunately, nicotine has been found to be linked to hair loss. The Times of India notes that nicotine narrows your blood vessels, slowing fresh hair growth down. Blood vessels are key to growing hair faster and thicker, according to the Massachusetts General Hospital. Smoking electronic cigarettes may slow down your hair growth, speeding up the effects of balding and thinning."

Skin Disease

Dermatologists weigh in. In an article in *Fitness* magazine it's reported that all smoking is bad for the skin. The habit deprives your skin of oxygen and constricts blood flow. It affects circulation and breaks down the necessary nutrients like collagen and Vitamin C. One thing is certain, as reported by dermatologist Karen Soika of The Cosmetic Medic and RealSelf contributor Joel Schlessinger, "It's difficult to say what the long-term effects of prolonged use might be. Because the chemicals are the same, it's highly likely that using a vaporizer will still do the same amount of damage to your skin. Plus, because you're still puckering your lips, you'll still develop deep lines and wrinkles around the mouth."

Confirmed also by Dr. Raja is that "the nicotine in vaping liquids dehydrates your skin, so you can get premature wrinkles and very dry skin, which don't look good. In addition to skin aging, too, vaping can also delay wound healing. So, if you get a paper cut, that paper cut is going to stick with you." But even worse: The search has also found that nicotine use is linked to chronic skin conditions like acne and psoriasis, and skin cancers such as squamous cell carcinoma and melanoma, as well as oral cancer. So, if the experts are right, and nicotine is at the root of these conditions, one can assume that vaping nicotine will produce the same devastating results.

Smoking itself, whether it's traditional cigarettes or e-cigarettes, ups your chances for skin cancers, such as squamous cell carcinoma. It's been reported that 75% of oral cancers occur in smokers. And, as mentioned, you can practically guarantee changes to your teeth as the vaping liquids will start to yellow your teeth; the more you do it the worse it will get, but count on inflammation as well. As it begins to affect your organs so it will your gums. Excessive vaping may eventually lead to tooth loss.

Autoimmune Disease

Here is the story of a patient at New York's Mt. Sinai who was being treated by a gastroenterologist for irritable bowel disease. In the process of trying to determine whether the patient had ulcerative colitis or Crohn's disease, among the multitude of tests, biopsies, colonoscopies and blood work, a question was asked:

"Are you by any chance a smoker who has recently quit?" The patient was astounded as she had quit cigarette smoking earlier that year. The doctor went on to describe a hunch theory regarding autoimmune disease, explaining that there is some evidence to suggest that in people who may be pre-disposed to an autoimmune disease, if they add a toxin to their body for some time, and then remove it, that patient's autoimmune response will be turned on in a different way than other people; in fact, in such a way that it doesn't turn off. Interestingly enough, when certain medications did not work for this patient, she was put on a mild nicotine patch and went into remission for nine months. It should be added that this was not a formal study. We have no idea whether this patient would have gotten IBD had she not smoked or even kept smoking. But think about the toxin, nicotine. Our bodies' natural response is to fight it. And with so little research about vaping, it stands to reason that many conditions common to cigarette smoking are just a 10-year study (or less) away from being found to come from e-cigarettes and the vessels, liquids, and chemicals that become vapor and make their way into the lungs and organs of the vaper.

Additionally, because vaping itself is new, oftentimes even doctors are unaware of how it may be conflagrating a diagnosis or prescription. One group at the same hospital in New York reports that they've admitted a couple of patients with pneumonitis thinking it might be from the meds they prescribed for gastrointestinal issues, only to learn that it was from surreptitious vaping. They write, "This patient was self-treating/exacerbating an anxiety disorder with cannabis vaping. It was extremely confusing to all of us." Though the patient recovered his pulmonary function will likely never be 100%.

In terms of lifelong issues, patients experiencing VTDs are likely to suffer from PTVD (post traumatic vape disorder).

For now, here is a quick and dirty guide to VTDs and/or their treatment:

EVALI:

The name given by the CDC that stands for e-cigarette, or vaping, product use-associated lung injury.

EXTREME, SEVERE, PULMONARY AND RESPIRATORY SYMTONS PRESENTING AS PNEUMONIA:

May require repeated lung treatments due to vaping and may be lifelong. Many patients first experience gastrointestinal symptoms like nausea, vomiting and diarrhea prior to respiratory symptoms. Might require intubation and being put on a ventilator indefinitely plus steroids.

ECMO:

Use of specialized ventilators as dialysis for the lungs, taking blood out of the body. Recycles blood gases by removing carbon dioxide and replacing oxygen in the lungs for lung recovery.

POPCORN LUNG (BRONCHIOLITIS OBLITERANS):

This disease damages and scars the lung tissue permanently and is irreversible once it constricts the airways. Symptoms include chronic coughing, shortness of breath, flu-like symptoms and fever. Popcorn lung is due to chemicals found in marijuana and some e-cigarettes.

LUNG TRANSPLANT:

This is the ultimate and most serious possibility for damages to lungs due to vaping.

RELAPSE:

Occurs frequently between the 5th and 55th day after initial hospital admission.

Definite reasons are still not known but possible explanations include lung weakness, infections, ineffective tapering of steroids.

VAPE TONGUE:

A sensation of thick coating on the tongue that blocks the ability to taste.

NEUROLOGICAL VAPE EFFECTS:

- 71% higher risk of stroke.

- 59% higher risk of heart attack or angina.

- 40% higher risk of heart disease.

SEIZURES AND CONVULSIONS:

These are known symptoms of nicotine toxicity.

ADDICTION AND BRAIN ALTERATION:

Nicotine causes an interruption in brain development making it harder to concentrate and learn. It affects mood, causes impulsivity and changes in the brain associated with addiction.

PERMAMENT DISABILTY:

Vaping can cause strokes, seizures, and permanent lung injury. As of December, 2019 confirmed hospitalizations have risen to 2409.

DEATH:

Vaping can cause death. As of December, 2019, 52 people have died due to vaping-related injuries in the U.S. and this figure continues to rise.

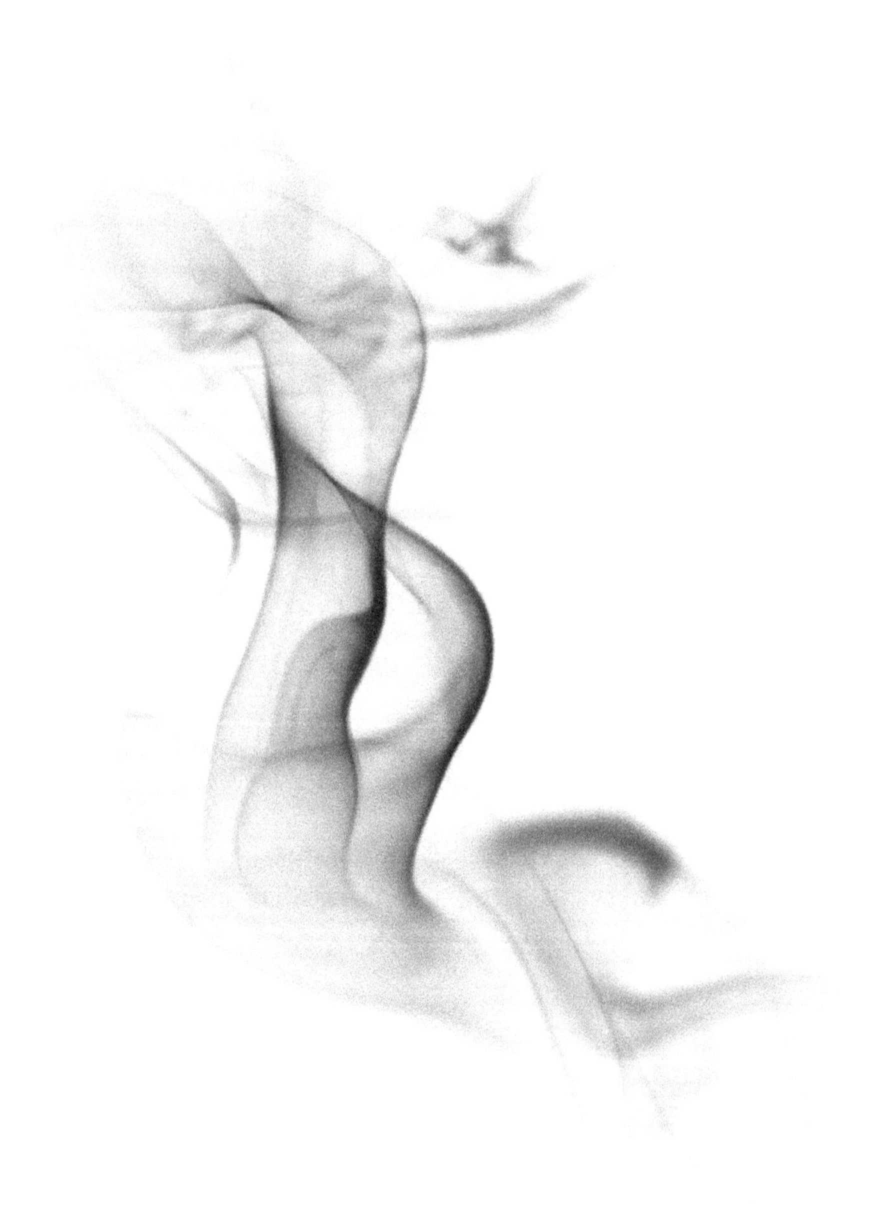

CHAPTER 9

The Vapes of Wrath

As evidence of vaping- and Juul-related illnesses and deaths became clear, the pressure on Juul to make changes became overwhelming, specifically as relates to teens and marketing to minors.

In November of 2018, Juul pledged to discontinue some flavors at retail outlets and shut down social media accounts ahead of an expected FDA crackdown. Initially, their announced plan seemed aggressive. Yet under scrutiny, their proposed "self-regulation" was seen as anemic. In an article on www.wired.com former FDA commissioner Scott Gottlieb called for stronger actions across the board when it came to all e-cigarette manufacturers in order to "reverse the trend" of youth use of vaping products which he categorized as epidemic.

Juul said they will no longer accept retail orders on fruity flavorings but will not eliminate menthol, mint and tobacco pods. And there are some confusing conditions. In the fine print, it appears that if the shop selling the flavors adheres to only serving customers who are 21 and older, they may get the flavors back. The stores will have to comply with certain other restrictions. Who will be creating those restrictions? Juul! Can you say...Loopholes?

This first and weak concession is so disturbing on a number of levels. First, consider that it completely dismisses the health effects we've seen on our young adults, a population we still consider our youth. Think of the popularity on college campuses, and of course the easy access for the under-21 set. And while Juul proposed to shut their U.S.-based Facebook and Instagram accounts, the "devil was out of the box" as evidenced by users' own social media accounts spreading the word. Remember the hashtags? Well, between the products' launch in June of 2015 and the company's ceasing of their own social media marketing at the time of the *Wired* article, over a quarter of a million posts appeared. What's happened since? We've learned from the same group at Stanford studying the Juul that the rate of community posting has accelerated quickly and markedly; in fact, it has doubled to over half a million. The takeaway is that no matter what Juul does now in terms of social media, their advertising can't be stopped as it has a youth life of its own.

Additionally, as reported in *The New York Times,* the statements from Juul executives at the time were seen as obligatory not voluntary. CEO of Juul Labs Kevin Burns is quoted as saying, "Our intent was never to have youth use Juul, but intent is not enough. The numbers are what matter and the numbers tell us underage use of e-cigarettes is a problem."

Wow. It's hard not to be reminded of those 1974 congressional hearings and a parade of tobacco executives robotically stating, "I don't believe nicotine is addictive." Kids, parents, educators, physicians, attorneys, regulators, scientists and, in fact, everyone in the country is asking, 'You didn't intend to market to kids? What adult wants to smoke gummy bears or fruit loops?' It's hard not to be outraged and offended by the condescension and the lies. It's also sad to note that no moral directive, just as with Big Tobacco, took hold, if it even has, until the company had no choice. Not much choice when teens are in medically-induced comas for pulmonary issues or a double lung transplant.

Furthermore, Juul had hired lobbyists in 2017. Despite pledging that their product was not intended for youth use, they accelerated spending after Altria spent $13 billion to acquire a stake in the company. As reported in Wired, data from the FDA, which prompted increased scrutiny from Gottlieb, shows that between 2017 and 2018 the number of kids who vaped grew 75 percent, with more than two million middle- and high-school students using e-cigs in 2017. The company is still lobbying heavily and faces a barrage of lawsuits about addicting users to nicotine.

"After an April 2018 inquiry from the Food and Drug Administration about its marketing, Juul pledged to spend $30 million over the next three years on youth smoking prevention and to support Tobacco 21, a national campaign aimed at raising the minimum age for tobacco and nicotine sales in the US. In June of that year, the company vowed to stop using models in its social media ads and to work with social media companies to remove offending posts and accounts."

The FDA acknowledged that it had been slow to catch up to the problem. In September of 2018 it gave Juul and other e-cigarette makers 60 days to submit plans showing and proving that they could correct the problem of minors having access to their products. Juul also vowed to improve online verification, shipping of bulk orders to minors and other restrictions on the number of pods that could be purchased. They also offered to ask the social media companies to help them police posts that might in some way draw in underage users.

Under the heading of "too little too late," one of the most astounding facts to come out in recent months, concluded by the National Academies and reported by the *Times* and in the Netflix documentary, is that as it turns out, teenagers who use these devices may be at higher risk and are even likelier to use real cigarettes in the future.

Despite this, and despite their promises, it seems that between November of 2018 and November of 2019, Juul dug their heels in and actually ramped up their opposition to the changing climate. In July of 2019 they geared up for a major fight over local bans on vaping around the country. As reported by Politico, Juul had been at odds with San Francisco, the city where they essentially began and where they held their headquarters, since 2017, when the city banned all flavors. Despite a contentious and financially-rich fight, the city instituted a ban on all vaping products. The fight continues, but it's expected that until the FDA has a chance to study and determine considerations that best serve the public health, the ban will remain in effect.

Juul continues to insist that they want to work with "policymakers, lawmakers, FDA regulators, educators and parents on youth education and prevention." They insist that they want to be part of the solution without exactly acknowledging their part in the problem. Ironically, as Juul's wallet grows fatter and the public grows sicker, the battle almost exactly mirrors what happened with Big Tobacco versus consumers. The article in *Wired* suggests that it must make for an interesting platform crevice, between Juul's public face where they must look contrite and willing to help solve the youth consumption problem, and the boardroom face, where they must placate and assure investors who've spent sizable sums banking on the youth consumption continuation, that the company will remain whole.

Those who support Juul are not necessarily on the side of vaping but against coercion. As is often the case with "choice" items in history, there is an ongoing debate about government interference and overregulation versus personal freedoms. Yet these arguments are often strongest when it comes to debates over what is informally known as "victimless crimes," such as gambling or prostitution. While no one would argue that these are, essentially, victimless, and in fact could quite easily argue for the negative domino effect that each creates, they don't translate to bodily harm in the instant, linear way that smoking does. And even with cigarette smoking, as we've mentioned, the harm is successive and long-term. So, in light of the progress that's been reversed regarding teen smoking and the epidemic of vaping that would seem to be grooming a new generation of smokers, the city of San Francisco remains firm that more studies need to be done and more regulations need to be in place to protect the public, and especially minors. Other municipalities are following their lead. States such as **Illinois, New Jersey** and **Delaware** are considering legislation, including bans on sales of all youth-friendly e-cigarettes, but some states already have bans in place.

As reported in *Time* magazine, **Michigan** has drastically curtailed sales of any product with a flavor other than tobacco and has plans to restrict packaging words like "clean, safe, and healthy." The ban is time-limited and being fought by retailers.

New York has implemented a statewide ban on most flavored nicotine products; however, just as it was about to take effect, it was put on hold.

Massachusetts declared a public health emergency in September of 2019. A new law, set to take effect in June of 2020, will have severe restrictions but is not a blanket ban. In **Rhode Island**, a total ban on vaping was in place for 4 months and extensions are currently being debated.

Montana, Oregon, Washington and California have all banned some version of flavored e-cigarettes or cannabis vaping products.

The Public Health Law Center in **Minnesota** publishes the following under their article, "Juul and the Guinea Pig Generation":

"Use of e-cigarettes by youth is strongly associated with use of other tobacco products, including conventional cigarettes and other burned tobacco products. Research has found that youth who use e-cigarettes are more likely to go on to use other tobacco products, including conventional cigarettes." With regards to regulations, they address the following question:

Q: Is Juul subject to federal, state, or local regulation?

A combination of federal, state, and local policy options can be pursued to strengthen regulation of Juul and other e-cigarettes. The Public Health Law Center's website has multiple resources on e-cigarette regulation. Prominent policy options that can help prevent initiation and use of Juul and other electronic cigarettes and e-liquids include:

Sales

Prohibiting sales of e-cigarettes and e-liquids to persons under 21;

Restricting locations of sales to adult-only licensed retailers that are off-limits to persons under 21;

Prohibiting sales of flavored e-cigarettes and e-liquids or restricting sales of such products to licensed retailers that do not allow persons under 21 to purchase or enter at any time;

Prohibiting the sale of e-cigarettes and e-liquids with a nicotine concentration over a certain amount (e.g., over 40 mg/ml);

Prohibiting direct shipping of online orders of e-cigarettes and e-liquids to consumers (e.g., allowing online orders to be shipped only to licensed distributors or retailers); and

Restricting and monitoring shipments by strengthening age verification, shipment, and enforcement policies.

Use

Amending school policies and state and local smoke-free or tobacco-free workplace laws by adding or updating definitions and policy language, as needed, to prohibit e-cigarette use in settings where smoking is prohibited.

Marketing

Addressing false or misleading claims through use of state consumer protection and/or unfair trade practice laws; and

Placing limits on advertising, to the extent permitted by law.

Pricing

Prohibiting all free and nominal price sampling of e-cigarettes and e-liquids, regardless of whether they purport to contain no nicotine;

Prohibiting discounting of products;

Imposing state excise taxes of e-cigarettes and e-juices to achieve parity (be on par)

with taxation of other tobacco products and to keep taxes at a high enough level to discourage youth initiation and continuation of use.

Ingredient disclosure and/or lab testing

Requiring manufacturers to report lab tests to verify all active ingredients and their concentration levels.

While the FDA has full authority to take all these requested actions, or a more comprehensive action, stringently enforcing premarket review by ordering every Juul product off the market entirely until the agency has reviewed the products and authorized their marketing, it has yet to do so.

For a complete list of the latest regulations by state and city, check out this site by the Public Health Law Center. https://www.publichealthlawcenter.org/resources/us-e-cigarette-regulations-50-state-review

As of December, 2019, 50 states and the District of Columbia have implemented laws regarding sales of e-cigarettes to minors. Some define a minor as 18 or 19, others as 21, but by July of 2020 the minimum age to purchase e-cigarettes will be age 20. Just to get an idea of regulations, here are three states with recent laws targeting sales to minors:

VERMONT

What restrictions are in place for retail or youth access?

Sale/distribution of tobacco substitutes to persons under age 21 prohibited.

7 Vt. Stat. Ann § 1003(a) (2019)

Purchase/possession of tobacco substitutes by persons under age 21 prohibited.

7 Vt. Stat. Ann. § 1005(a)(1) (2019)

Self-service displays restricted to locations inaccessible to persons under age 21 years. 7 Vt. Stat. Ann. § 1003(c)(2) (2019)

No person under the age of 16 years may sell tobacco substitutes. 7 Vt. Stat. Ann. § 1002(f) (2019)

FLORIDA

What restrictions are in place for retail or youth access?

Sale/distribution of nicotine dispensing devices or nicotine products to persons under age 18 prohibited. Fla. Stat. § 877.112(2)-(3) (2019)

Possession of nicotine dispensing devices or nicotine products by persons under age 18 prohibited. Fla. Stat. § 877.112(6) (2019)

Self-service displays of nicotine products or nicotine dispensing devices prohibited in places accessible to persons under 18 years except sales made through vending machine with lockout device controlled by retailer. Fla. Stat. § 877.112(11)(12) (2019)

TEXAS

What restrictions are in place for retail or youth access?

Sale/distribution of e-cigarettes and distribution/redemption of coupons for e-cigarettes to persons under age 21 is prohibited (unless purchaser is at least 18 and has U.S. or state military id card). Tex. Health & Safety Code Ann.§§ 161.082, 161.087 (2019) (increased MLSA effective September 1, 2019) (publicly accessible version not yet updated)

Purchase/possession/use of e-cigarettes by persons under age 21 years prohibited unless at least 18 with a U.S. or state military id card. Tex. Health & Safety Code Ann.§ 161.252 (2019) (increased MLSA effective September 1, 2019) (publicly accessible version not yet updated)

Self-service/vending sales of e-cigarettes restricted to locations inaccessible to persons under age 21. Tex. Health & Safety Code Ann. § 161.086 (2019) (increased MLSA effective September 1, 2019) (publicly accessible version not yet updated)

Retailers of e-cigarette delivery sales must register with the state, verify, at time of purchase and at delivery, that the purchaser is over 21 years of age, include a notice about the prohibition on selling e-cigarettes to minors, and file certain information about the purchaser with the comptroller. Tex. Health & Safety Code Ann. § 161.452(c) (2019) (increased MLSA effective September 1, 2019) (publicly accessible version not yet updated)

In September of 2019 President Trump announced plans to remove all youth-friendly flavored vaping products, including mint and menthol. This proved to be controversial, receiving praise from those in public health but loud protests from vaping industry organizations. As weeks went by, it seemed the protesters were more persuasive and no official policy was crafted or installed into law. A meeting was held at the White House to discuss and debate the pros and cons. While Trump conceded that there was an epidemic at the level of a public health crisis, and this was validated by public health and medical experts, Trump raised concerns regarding the black market, among other issues, and seemed to back off the proposed flavor ban but did promise that the age to buy e-cigarettes will be raised to 21.

In terms of removing flavored products, even executives from the different e-cigarette companies were not in sync. Rival companies to Juul accused them of less than altruistic motives for removing the flavored pods, citing their 70% market share that would grow if the smaller company's profits dwindled due to lack of flavored offerings. As reported by Time.com, NJOY CEO Ryan Nivakoff actually accused Juul of trying to "wait out" the failure of its competitors.

Also discussed was the ongoing debate about whether e-cigarettes even help with their professed target audiences' desire or need to quit traditional smoking.

As reported by the *New York Times,* Mitt Romney, who was seated to the right of Mr. Trump, noted that "most adults are not using flavors" and that those products were targeting and addicting youth vapers.

"Putting out cotton candy flavor and unicorn poop flavor, this is a kid product," Mr. Romney said. "We have to put the kids first." Vaping executives begged to differ, insisting that adults are using flavored e-cigarettes to quit smoking. But Romney countered, "Utah is a Mormon state, and half the kids in high school are vaping," he said.

In the first half of 2019, Juul spent nearly $2 million, funded 24 lobbyists, and contributed approximately $200 grand to favorable political candidates. In March of that year, the head of the FDA, Dr. Scott Gottlieb, stepped down several months before the end of his term, stating that he wanted to spend more time with his family. In the months since, he has continued to warn the public about vaping and recently told CNBC he believed the government needed to regulate cannabis products, referring to reports of 450 possible cases and five deaths from a mysterious lung disease linked to vaping. Many of these patients reported combining nicotine and THC, though some used only nicotine. By November, the former commissioner was calling for a full ban on pod-based e-cigarettes. As he said in an interview with www.statenews.com "he's done playing nice guy." As we now know, the number of deaths in the U.S. as a result of vaping has risen to 60.

Beginning in September, Dr. Gottlieb tweeted *@scottgottliebmd:*

Another policy consideration was to remove cartridge based products from market, which are the kinds of cheap, fashionable products favored by kids; and allow the open tank vaping systems to continue to be sold in mostly adult vaping stores that do better job limiting kid access.

And again:

If I seem personally upset by this turn of events today, it's because I've watched Juul actively work to try and thwart public health efforts to get better regulation over products that we know are hurting children.

And further:

Another tragic reality of these events is that these products, properly regulated, could potentially help millions of currently addicted adult smokers quit cigarettes. That opportunity will be slowed now as a result of actions required to stem youth epidemic Juul helped create.

And in November, echoing the concerns of Juul's rivals:

Perhaps Juul says it supports the flavor ban because they may be one of the few products left on the market after it takes effect. Having been the key driver of this youth epidemic, it's adult vape stores that will bear the brunt of the flavor ban.

And in November of 2019,

It's very clear that Juul can't keep their products out of the hands of kids. What's driving the youth use is primarily Juul. You've hooked a lot of kids," he added. "Kids now, it's become sort of fashionable and they like the form and fashion of this product. It could be that this product can't exist on the market anymore."

The New York Times notes that in an interview on CNBC, Dr. Gottlieb also said he thought the administration was legitimately concerned about the economic effects on the thousands of vape shops that have sprung up around the country and predicted that the businesses might get a carve-out from any initiative aimed at restricting flavors. Mr. Trump and his advisers have mentioned the jobs created by the industry in earlier remarks. As of December 2019, no official ban or announcement has been made and the issue remains unresolved. Politico reports that Trump is being influenced by "vaping voters" and is caught in the middle. Even wife Melania is concerned about the youth vaping epidemic. She tweeted the latest CDC data in September: "It's our responsibility as parents to understand the dangers that come from vaping. Our Administration supports the removal of flavored e-cigarettes from stores until they're approved by @US_FDA."

In some ways, September of 2019 seems to have been a turning point. First, Juul replaced their CEO with a tobacco executive. As reported in *Financial Times*, Kevin Burns was out and KC Crosthwaite, the very definition of giant tobacco, Altria's tobacco chief growth officer, took the helm of Juul. This was less than a year after Altria acquired Juul Labs. Concurrently, Juul has also said it has a new marketing strategy: It will suspend all TV, print and digital ads and will stop some of its lobbying efforts.

In response, Nancy Brown, head of the American Heart Association, said the installation of Mr. Crosthwaite showed that Juul was "fully embracing its identity as a tobacco company that prioritizes profits over public health".

Others are also not swayed. In a CNN Business report Tim Hubbard, assistant professor of management in the business school at Notre Dame: "Bringing in a traditional tobacco executive who knows how to market and manage government relationships with deadly products matches the firm's needs." Hubbard continued, "We can expect a change to traditional tobacco strategies as the company tries to adjust to a new reality."

One anti-smoking group said no one should be lulled into thinking that Juul has changed.

Matthew Myers, president of the Campaign for Tobacco-Free Kids warns that no one should be lulled into thinking that Juul has changed. "The youth e-cigarette epidemic has gone from bad to worse, and 5 million kids now use e-cigarettes. Juul's announcement today is aimed at repairing its image and protecting its profits, not at solving this crisis. This announcement strips away any doubt about Juul. It is Big Tobacco."

Finally, in early January of 2020, the Trump administration did put some bans in effect, but these bans are seen as a retreat from the "previous, stricter proposal" as reported in the *LA Times,* and though a move in the right direction, considered soft by those on the tragic side of the epidemic of addicted youth. One reason the move is disappointing is that it does nothing to address the lure of tobacco and menthol flavors, which we know are highly appealing, just as they were to smokers of traditional cigarettes. These can continue to be marketed. Ultimately, with no full vaping ban in place, these laws do nothing to address those already addicted.

And, because the flavors were previously introduced and became part of youth culture, you can bet they will be available in an even more destructive way, on the black market. We have Juul to thank for this as well. Alex Axar, Trump's Secretary of Health and Human Services, stated in an article for Business Insider, "We will not stand idly by as these products become an on-ramp to combustible cigarettes or nicotine addiction for a generation of youth."

https://www.businessinsider.com/trump-flavor-ban-vapes-e-cigarettes-sweet-fruit-report-2019-11

We can only hope that the costs to Juul, which are becoming somewhat significant, continue to do so. Their new CEO has pledged to cut $1 billion in costs. This will include cutting approximately 650 jobs. And these are said to be significantly in the marketing department. Calling it a "reboot," or "reset," changes will be made to fix the company's image and "shrinking valuation." As of November of 2019 Reuters reports that Altria's investment has devalued by a third. Of course, keeping things in perspective, this "significant devaluation" in financial worth takes Juul's net worth from $28.5 billion down to $24 billion. Its stock was valued at roughly $230 a share, around the recent share price of Apple and about $100 more than the price of eBay and PayPal stock combined.

No doubt the patients and families embracing a lifetime of health ramifications would be unmoved.

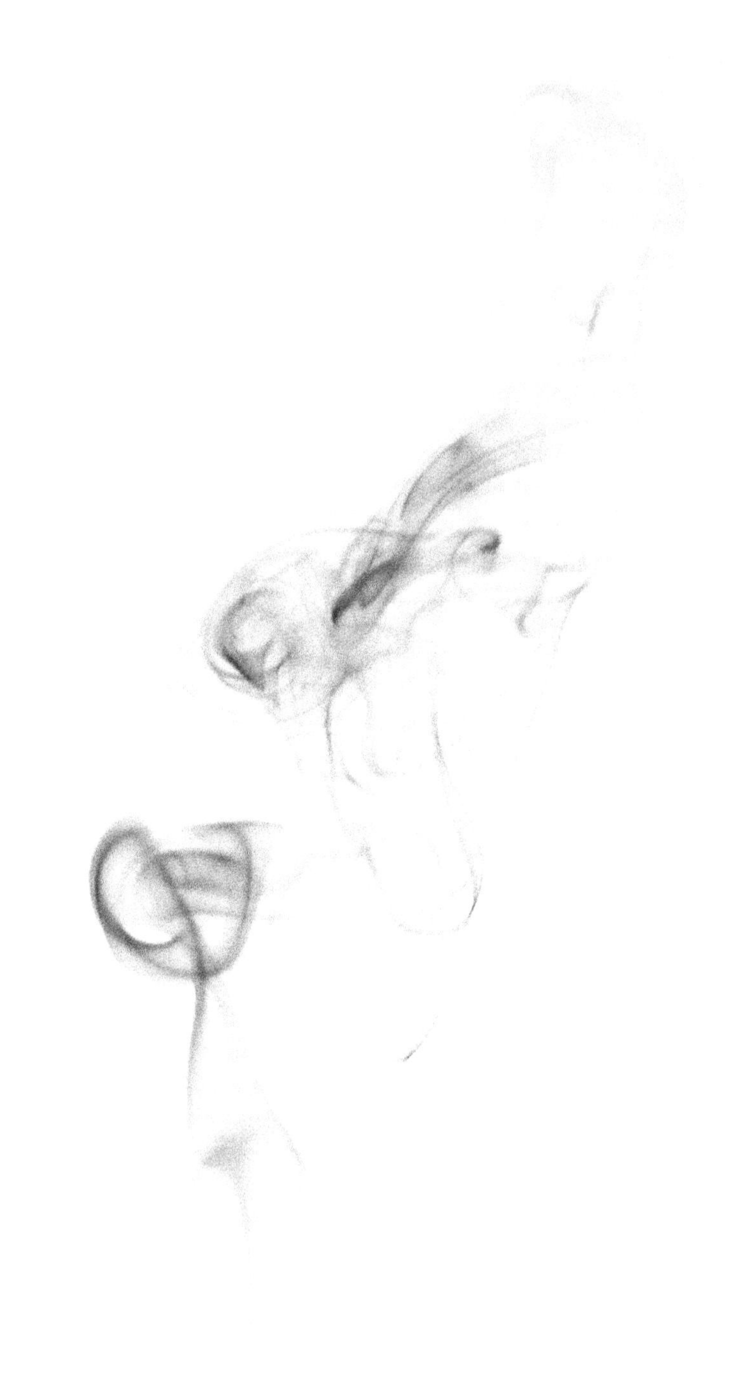

CHAPTER 10

PTVD: Post Traumatic Vaping Disorder

A great reflection of the country's climate is often seen in the art and entertainment world. Consider this exchange of dialogue on Showtime's hit show *Shameless* between main character and young adult "Lip," a cigarette smoker, and first his brother, Ian, and then his boss. References to Freddy are about his newborn son.

IAN: You smell like caramel.

LIP: Got one of these vapor things. Trying to quit.

IAN: Aren't these things worse for you?

LIP: Yeah you know they market these things to kids? Bastards would have one of these things in Freddy's hands if he could hold more than a bottle.

LIP: I think I'm addicted.

BOSS: You and every other junior high school girl. What is it, Mint? Cotton Candy? Those marketing dudes are criminal.

And on *The Simpsons:*

In a 2015 episode, vaping pervades Springfield, with all major characters – even baby Maggie and Grampa Abe – blowing rings.

The show then mocks the relative availability of E-cigs to children, by having convenience store owner Apu try and sell Bart on flavored vapes, saying, "It's not kid's stuff. Now do you want bubblegum or tropical melon flavor?"

And on the show *True Detective,* two main characters, Ani and Ray, discuss e-cigarettes. Ray says, "I tried one once. It felt like it was smoking me. A real cigarette wouldn't make you feel like that. Maybe it's just too close to sucking a robot's dick! I don't know." But what's even more significant about the episode is that we never, ever see Ani vaping in any episode again. In fact, three episodes later she is back to cigarette smoking.

Fox News reports that the FDA released its first anti-vaping television ads on ESPN, targeting teens as part of its "The Real Cost" Youth e-cigarette Prevention Campaign. The ads, titled "Magic," feature street magician Julius Dein turning teens' vapes into cigarettes. Dein's YouTube channel has almost 800,000 subscribers, his Twitter has over 80,000 followers and he's appeared in videos with several celebrities, according to the FDA.

"Did you know that if you vape, you are more likely to start smoking cigarettes?" Dein asks a stunned group of young people after the e-cigarette in one teen's hand disappears and is replaced by a traditional cigarette.

"It's not magic, it's statistics."

In a TED Talk by Suchitra Krishnan-Sarin, a bio behavioral scientist, vaping is explained and warnings to parents are stern. As she says, "Our health, the health of our children and our future generations is far too valuable to let it go up in smoke — or even in aerosol."

Have you seen the latest ads from Michael R. Bloomberg, who is running for president? Not only has he championed scrutiny and limitations on vaping, calling it a health crisis of epidemic proportions, but his latest ad points at his accomplishments in safeguarding public health and creating laws to keep our youth from addiction, and features a full screen shot of a Juul package as an accompaniment.

It seems, if the public is to be educated and warned about the dangers of e-cigarettes and vaping, and educated and warned about the epidemic of use by youth, utilizing the media and social media, the very vehicles that exposed the country to Juul and other vape companies, may make the most sense and have the greatest impact.

Finally, as of early 2020, here is what we know for sure:

In the United States, 59 confirmed deaths linked to vaping and a total of 2602 hospitalized patients with respiratory illnesses linked to same. The CDC categorizes this as an "outbreak."

Of those who were sickened or died, approximate percentages by age are below:

16% were under 18 years old.

38% were 18 to 24 years old.

24% were 25 to 34 years old.

23% were 35 or older.

If we do a bit of math, that means that over 50% at least were college-age or younger, still developing physically, mentally, and emotionally.

Additional data regarding youth use reveals that "more than one in four high school students in the U.S. use e-cigarettes. Most who vape, do so daily."

The National Institute on Drug Abuse report of vaping teens states that "vaping prevalence has more than doubled for 8th, 10th, and 12th graders." (grades surveyed)

A New York survey found that 1 in 15 middle schoolers smoked e-cigarettes. The growth rate nationally for middle schoolers vaping was nearly 50% in 2019. (CDC)

With Juul dominating the market at approximately 70%, many teen vapers simply refer to it as JuulING, not smoking.

On their website, www.Juul.com, Juul states that they have ongoing actions to combat underage use, including Retail Access Control Standards (RACS), Online Age Verification, Track and Trace, Tobacco 21, Secret Shopper programs, and technology-based solutions.

Additionally, they commit to ways that they are limiting appeal. These include restricting flavors and removing existing social media.

An article in usnews.com pointedly asks, "Too Little Too Late?" Many who've been covering the "vaping crisis" for years report constant pushback from Juul over the past several years, and that the company only made changes when public outcry might damage their image more than the loss of sales associated with the changes. For instance, *The New York Times* reports that Juul refused to sign a pledge not to market to teens as part of a lawsuit settlement. And former executives and employees point out that the company was "never just about helping adult smokers." These sentiments are corroborated in legal filings and social media archives.

Now, there is an overall sentiment, in light of the increase in youth use, that Juul is only doing what they have to because "they got caught."

Perhaps the saddest endnote to the controversy, the horrific illnesses and deaths notwithstanding, comes from a comment by Connie Pechmann, a marketing professor at the University of California-Irvine in usnews.com. Pechmann has studied the link between youth smoking rates and cigarette advertising. She says

Juul is responsible for hooking a new generation of young users, just like Big Tobacco did decades earlier. "The rise of vaping and popularity of Juul," she says, "threaten [all] the gains made by hooking a new generation on nicotine. Data shows teens who vape are four times more likely to try cigarettes, and Juul says a single pod can contain the same nicotine strength as a full pack of 20 cigarettes. Smoking was almost gone. Now we're back to square one."

Statutory Vape: the act of selling or providing e-cigarette materials to those under the age of 18.

If you or your family member want additional information and for the most current statistics and information about the e-cigarette crisis or where to get help, visit www.cdc.gov, www.fda.gov, https://e-cigarettes.surgeongeneral.gov, https://kidshealth.org and www.hive80.com and go to the Addiction hive.

Or, for legal information go to https://www.periscopegroup.com/injuries/Juul-vaping

If you'd like to tell us your story or talk to me about finding legal help for your Juul case, please email me at jennifer@statutoryyape.com.

If you or a loved one have respiratory symptoms possibly associated with vaping or e-cigarette use, visit your local ER immediately.

ACKNOWLEDGEMENTS

Writing an expose like this means you had a lot of dedicated people around you sharing your passion and working endless hours. Thank you to everyone who contributed. I always appreciate when I decide "we" are all going to do something like write this book and everyone gives it their all.

Thanks to Dr. Tsai for his passion and dedication to stopping vaping-related cases and to his endless hours treating patients. As a thoracic surgeon he has usually seen people 50 or older coming in for treatment. Now his patients are younger and younger and he is seeing a dramatic increase in high school students coming in with pulmonary complications due to vaping. One of his saddest cases in the last few months was an extremely healthy high school football player whose vaping phase led him to now live on a ventilator. Others need lung transplants or have reoccurring pulmonary issues.

Dr. Tsai is so passionate about stopping vaping, he started an educational program where he invites kids on rounds with him to see the carnage Juul has caused. Thank you, Dr. Tsai, for recognizing that this problem won't go away on its own. We hope other doctors follow suit and start being more active in the diagnosis and the treatment of vaping-related injuries.

Brooks Cutter, you are a rock star as a lawyer and a person. I have had the privilege of working with you for 25 years and I'm always in awe of your dedication to doing what's best for your clients and getting them great results. Keep up the good work on the e-cigarette and vaping settlements. We always enjoy working on these projects with you.

Much appreciation to my brother Mark for helping me to rewrite the Foreword of this book. You're a fantastic writer and an even better listener.

And to Jack Acosta. The best Musc a girl could have.

Biographies

Jennifer Banmiller is a successful serial entrepreneur and longtime consumer advocate. She has founded several companies, consumer websites and communities that illuminate unsafe products and unethical business practices in order to help inform and educate the general public.

She is the founder of Wingtip Communications and the legal consumer advocacy site www.periscopegroup.com. She authored the explosive expose *Crystal Mesh: How Addiction To Money turned Medical Device Makers, the FDA, and Doctors Into Street Dealers* (www.crystalmesh.com), which chronicled the horrors of vaginal mesh in the U.S. Most recently, she launched Hive80.com, a health and wellness community where consumers can access and share important answers to health questions, and engage with both their peers and the medical community to help the public lead more productive and happy lives. She wrote *Statutory Vape* to shine a light on the huge unfolding teenage public health crisis related to vaping, and to help teens, their families, and their friends understand the critical health issues before it is too late.

Wilson S. Tsai, MD graduated from the University of Medicine and Dentistry in New Jersey in 1999, but his journey started long before that. "Each of us makes life choices in response to events in our lives. I was motivated at an early age to become a doctor because of the feelings of helplessness that I felt when both my grandparents were battling cancer". Dr. Tsai knew his path was clear. He prepared himself early to be the best surgeon that he could be. His experiences in medical school confirmed his goal of devoting his life to treating patients with thoracic diseases.

Following medical school Dr. Tsai trained in general surgery at the Robert Wood Johnson Hospital in New Jersey. He then won an appointment to the fellowship program at the National Cancer Institute at the prestigious national Institute of Health in Bethesda, MD Following this fellowship, Dr. Tsai completed an additional cardiothoracic surgery fellowship at The University of Pittsburgh Medical Center specializing in thoracic surgery and remained at the medical center where he was honored to become a clinical instructor in minimally-invasive thoracic surgery. Also, he trained at the prestigious Memorial-Sloan Kettering Cancer Center as a thoracic fellow.

Dr. Tsai is the Co-Director of the Thoracic Surgical Program at John Muir Health, is board certified in thoracic surgery and has been a member of American Association for Thoracic Surgery since 1996. Dr. Tsai is committed to providing his patients with the latest advancements and treatment options. Since his appointment to the directorship at John Muir Health, he has established a minimally-invasive thoracic program that specializes in all aspects of benign and malignant esophageal and lung diseases. He had been granted a separate wing at John Muir Medical Center in Walnut Creek which boasts an impressive team of specially-trained nurses and a physician assistant who has had extensive experience in thoracic surgery at the Memorial Sloan Kettering Cancer Center. The dedicated thoracic floor enables patients to receive more focused care, and have shorter hospital stays. His John Muir thoracic program has drawn patients from as far as Nevada and Utah.

Dr. Tsai has been appointed as the Chair of the Thoracic Division at Sutter Eden Medical Center in Castro Valley. He has established a comprehensive thoracic program for Eden that serves patients from that part of the East Bay.

SOURCES/REFERENCES

Teague, Claude E. Jr.. Research Planning Memorandum on Some Thoughts About New Brands of Cigarettes for the Youth Market. 1973 February 02. Joe Camel Collection. Unknown. https://www.industrydocuments.ucsf.edu/docs/pspp0094

https://www.theguardian.com/society/2019/sep/10/Juul-is-the-new-big-tobacco-wave-of-lawsuits-signal-familiar-problems

https://www.bloomberg.com/news/features/2019-10-10/Juul-is-the-new-big-tobacco-as-anger-over-teen-vaping-escalates

https://truthinitiative.org/sites/default/files/media/files/2019/07/Examining-Juuls-role-in-the-youth-e-cigarette-epidemic.pdf

https://www.latimes.com/politics/story/2019-11-19/Juul-vaping-chemical-formulas-based-in-big-tobacco

https://www.mdanderson.org/publications/focused-on-health/is-vaping-safe-.h19-1592202.html

https://www.northcarolinahealthnews.org/2019/10/04/nc-hospital-spotted-mystery-vaping-injury-patterns-early-on/

https://www.nj.com/news/2019/08/9-hospitalized-with-mystery-illness-in-nj-after-vaping-heres-what-we-know.html

https://www.10tv.com/article/vaping-has-increased-700-ohio-schools-2016-2019-nov

https://www.cdph.ca.gov/Programs/CCDPHP/Pages/Vaping-Health-Advisory.aspx

https://www.edweek.org/ew/articles/2019/08/28/the-student-vaping-crisis-how-schools-are.html

https://www.fastcompany.com/90426336/im-the-mother-of-two-vaping-teens-Juul-should-pay-for-getting-kids-hooked

https://www.cdc.gov/tobacco/data_statistics/fact_sheets/youth_data/tobacco_use/index.htm

https://www.sciencenewsforstudents.org/article/explainer-nico-teen-brain

https://www.ncbi.nlm.nih.gov/pmc/articles/PMC3543069/

https://www.reddit.com/r/Juul/comments/bdpdys/why_dont_these_pods_have_warning_labels/

https://www.cnbc.com/2019/09/05/Juul-accused-of-illegally-advertising-vaping-as-a-way-to-quit-smoking.html

https://www.netflix.com/title/81059656

https://www.vox.com/2019/1/25/18194953/vape-Juul-e-cigarette-marketing

http://smokenders.com

https://www.insider.com/vape-juice-temporarily-desensitizing-peoples-taste-buds-2019-10

https://www.belgraviacentre.com/blog/new-study-may-explain-effect-of-e-cigarettes-on-hair-loss/

https://parade.com/931976/lisamulcahy/grossest-vaping-side-effects/

https://www.forbes.com/sites/kenrickcai/2019/07/18/teen-two-pod-a-day-Juul-addiction-caused-massive-stroke-lawsuit-vaping-e-cigarettes/#4c2bbfe16ace

https://www.fitnessmagazine.com/beauty/skin-care/everything-you-need-to-know-about-e-cigarettes-and-your-skin/

https://www.buzzfeednews.com/article/skbaer/teens-vaping-Juul-injury-warning-social-media

http://tobacco.stanford.edu/tobacco_main/publications/Hashtag_Juul_Project_7-22-19F.pdf

https://www.politico.com/story/2019/09/11/Juul-vaping-lobbying-washington-1491029

https://www.wired.com/story/Juuls-lobbying-could-send-its-public-image-up-in-smoke/

https://www.politico.com/story/2019/07/09/san-franciscos-electronic-cigarette-ban-Juul-1562168

https://www.ft.com/content/ef5c756c-dfe8-11e9-9743-db5a370481bc

https://www.cnn.com/2019/09/25/business/Juul-ceo-resigns/index.html

https://www.statnews.com/2019/11/12/gottlieb-ban-pod-based-e-cigarettes/

https://www.cnbc.com/2019/09/09/scott-gottlieb-federal-reckoning-needed-after-vaping-linked-deaths.html

https://socialunderground.com/2015/01/pax-ploom-origins-future-james-monsees/

https://nationalinterest.org/blog/buzz/are-e-cigarettes-sham-solution-or-excuse-98452

https://www.yahoo.com/news/ontario-teens-vaping-injury-consistent-050116188.html?.tsrc=fauxdal

https://uihc.org/health-topics/family-guide-ecmo

https://www.mayoclinic.org/tests-procedures/tracheostomy/about/pac-20384673

https://www.thedailybeast.com/this-surgeon-has-treated-30-people-for-exploding-e-cigarettes

https://www.washingtonpost.com/local/trafficandcommuting/with-little-faa-direction-vaping-devices-add-to-fire-dangers-on-planes/2019/10/03/8de85be0-ca8d-11e9-a1fe-ca46e8d573c0_story.html

https://www.johnsonbecker.com/product-liability/e-cigarette-explosion-lawsuit/?gclid=EAIaIQobChMI0JrTl_yo5gIVCmyGCh3ttwhXEAAYASAAEgLl7PD_BwE

https://www.fda.gov/safety/recalls-market-withdrawals-safety-alerts/urgent-voluntary-product-recall-vuse-vibe-power-units

https://www.nbcnews.com/health/health-news/battery-behind-dangerous-deadly-e-cigarette-explosions-n1032901

https://time.com/5685936/state-vaping-bans/

https://time.com/5737372/trump-vaping-meeting/

https://www.nytimes.com/2019/11/22/health/trump-vaping.html

https://www.politico.com/news/2019/11/27/vaping-voters-trump-e-cigarettes-074212

https://vaping360.com/lifestyle/vaping-in-tv-shows-movies/#true-detective-s2-e2

https://www.youtube.com/watch?v=a63t8r70QN0

https://www.publichealthlawcenter.org/sites/default/files/resources/Juul-and-the-Guinea-Pig-Generation-2018.pdf

https://www.cdc.gov/tobacco/basic_information/e-cigarettes/severe-lung-disease.html

https://www.cnbc.com/2019/09/12/cdc-says-teen-vaping-surges-to-more-than-1-in-4-high-school-students.html

https://www.nytimes.com/2019/09/18/health/vaping-teens-e-cigarettes.html

https://www.heart.org/en/news/2019/08/16/amid-an-epidemic-of-school-vaping-a-search-for-solutions

https://www.nytimes.com/2019/11/23/health/Juul-vaping-crisis.html

https://www.usnews.com/news/healthiest-communities/articles/2019-10-11/are-Juul-countermeasures-too-little-too-late

https://www.dailymail.co.uk/news/article-7717187/22-years-old-brink-death-vaping.html

https://www.latimes.com/politics/story/2020-01-02/trump-administration-retreats-from-vaping-flavor-ban

https://www.dailymail.co.uk/health/article-7786593/U-S-vaping-related-deaths-rise-52-hospitalizations-2-409.html

https://www.yahoo.com/lifestyle/harvard-researchers-discover-potential-asthmainducing-toxins-in-Juul-pods-150024850.html?guccounter=1

https://www.drugs.com/search.php?searchterm=Juul

STAY CURRENT

The vaping story has much longer legs and will go on far after the book is released. Please visit to www.statutoryvape.com f news, media and legal information.